O&M for Independent Living
Strategies for Teaching Orientation and Mobility to Older Adults

Nora Griffin-Shirley
and Laura Bozeman, *Editors*

AFB PRESS
American Foundation for the Blind

O&M for Independent Living: Strategies for Teaching Orientation and Mobility to Older Adults is copyright © 2016 by AFB Press, American Foundation for the Blind, 2 Penn Plaza, Suite 1102, New York, NY 10121. All rights reserved. No part of this work may be reproduced or transmitted in any form or by any means, electronic or mechanical, including photocopying and recording, or by any information storage or retrieval system, except as may be expressly permitted by the 1976 Copyright Act, or in writing from the publisher. Requests for permission should be addressed in writing to AFB Press, American Foundation for the Blind, 2 Penn Plaza, Suite 1102, New York, NY 10121.

Printed in the United States of America

Library of Congress Cataloging-in-Publication Data

O&M for independent living : strategies for teaching orientation and mobility to older adults / Nora Griffin-Shirley, PhD., and Laura Bozeman, PhD., (editors).
       pages cm
   Includes bibliographical references and index.
   ISBN 978-0-89128-676-9 (pbk. : alk. paper)—ISBN 978-0-89128-726-1 (online subscription)—ISBN 978-0-89128-727-8 (epub)—ISBN 978-0-89128-728-5 (mobi) 1. Blind—Orientation and mobility—Study and teaching. 2. Older people—Orientation and mobility—Study and teaching. I. Griffin-Shirley, Nora, 1954- editor. II. Bozeman, Laura, 1952- editor.
   HV1758.O16 2015
   362.4'18—dc23
                                                                    2015021242

The American Foundation for the Blind removes barriers, creates solutions, and expands possibilities so people with vision loss can achieve their full potential.

∞

It is the policy of the American Foundation for the Blind to use in the first printing of its books acid-free paper that meets the ANSI Z39.48 Standard. The infinity symbol that appears above indicates that the paper in this printing meets that standard.

CONTENTS

Acknowledgments v

About the Contributors vii

CHAPTER 1 **Vision Loss and Older Adults:** Considerations for the Orientation and Mobility Professional 1
Nora Griffin-Shirley and Laura Bozeman

CHAPTER 2 **Sensory Changes with Age:** Assessment Strategies for Older Adults with Visual Impairment 21
Laura Bozeman and Ken Bozeman

CHAPTER 3 **Modifying Orientation and Mobility Techniques for Older Adults with Visual Impairments** 45
Anita Page and Laura Bozeman

CHAPTER 4 **Orientation and Mobility Tools and Techniques** 79
James Scott Crawford

CHAPTER 5 **Environmental Adaptation and Modification** 141
Pat Crawford and Laura Bozeman

CHAPTER 6 **Importance of Exercise for Orientation and Mobility for Older Adults with Visual Impairments** 165
Laura Bozeman and Huan Zhang

CHAPTER 7 **Daily Living Skills and Orientation and Mobility:** Merging Skills to Enhance Life Satisfaction 179
Gretchen Good and Laura Bozeman

CHAPTER 8 **Fostering Collaboration among Professionals
Serving Older People with Vision Loss** 213
Rona Pogrund and Nora Griffin-Shirley

EPILOGUE **Current and Emerging Issues
for O&M Service Provision** 235
Nora Griffin-Shirley

Resources 245

Index 265

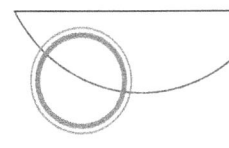

Acknowledgments

Our gratitude extends to the AFB Press editorial staff who encouraged us to write this book during our shared journey, starting with Natalie Hilzen, then George Abbot and Ellen Bilofsky.

In addition, the chapter authors have shown great perseverance in striving to meet deadlines, making suggested changes, and sharing their expertise and wisdom. It has been a joy and an honor to work with each one of them.

Finally, this book is dedicated to the older adults with vision impairments with whom we work and from whom we learn, the orientation and mobility specialists and other professionals who support the quality of life as defined by those individuals, and to our loved ones, James Michael Shirley, Buddy Holley, and Bonnie Bozeman.

—N. G.-S. and L.B.

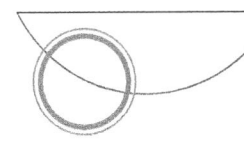

About the Contributors

EDITORS

Nora Griffin-Shirley, Ph.D., is professor and Coordinator of the Orientation and Mobility Program and TTU Graduate Certification Program in Sensory Impairments and Autism, and Director of the Virginia Murray Sowell Center for Research and Education in Sensory Disabilities at Texas Tech University. She is the co-author of *Prescriptions for Independence: Working with Older People Who Are Visually Impaired* and *Strength-Based Planning for Transitioning Students with Sensory Impairments*. Dr. Griffin-Shirley is also the co-author of book chapters, journal articles, and international conference presentations on the topics of orientation and mobility, strength-based planning, personnel preparation, and assistive technology competencies. She has previously served as treasurer, chair of the Orientation and Mobility Division, and board member of the Association for Education and Rehabilitation of the Blind and Visually Impaired.

Laura Bozeman, Ph.D., is Associate Professor and Director of Vision Studies at the School for Global Inclusion and Social Development at the University of Massachusetts, Boston. She has authored and co-authored book chapters and journal articles and presented internationally at conferences and workshops on the topics of low vision, orientation and mobility, personnel preparation, and vision assessment and has taught in the United States as well as in Taiwan, China, Saipan, Federated States of Micronesia, American Samoa, Australia, and New Zealand. Dr. Bozeman is the current chair of the Personnel Preparation Division and serves on the Executive Board of the Association for Education and Rehabilitation of the Blind and Visually Impaired.

CHAPTER AUTHORS

Ken Bozeman, Ph.D, Au.D., is an audiologist in private practice and at the Massachusetts Eye and Ear Infirmary in Boston.

James Scott Crawford, M.A., is a certified orientation and mobility specialist and certified low vision therapist and is an Instructional Supervisor at Affiliated Blind of Louisiana, Lafayette. He has been teaching orientation and mobility to individuals of all ages for over 25 years.

Pat Crawford, Ph.D., is Associate Director of the School of Planning, Design and Construction at Michigan State University. Dr. Crawford is a registered landscape architect whose accessibility work has been recognized by the Federal Access Board Regulatory Negotiation Committee's Recommendations for Accessibility Guidelines: Outdoor Developed Areas and the St. Louis chapter of the American Society of Landscape Architects. She has received service awards from the Missouri Governor's Council on Disability and was awarded the Missouri Rehabilitation Association President's Award and the Governor's award for quality and productivity.

Gretchen Good, Ph.D., is a senior lecturer in Rehabilitation and Public Health at Massey University, Palmerston North, New Zealand. Dr. Good is a certified vision rehabilitation therapist and orientation and mobility specialist who has authored or co-authored numerous journal articles on aging, vision loss, and quality of life of older adults with visual impairments and has published on the topics of children and visual impairment, disability and adoption, and disaster and disability. She serves on the elderly working group of the World Blind Union.

Anita Page, M.Ed., is Research Associate in Visual Impairment and O&M at the Virginia Murray Sowell Center for Research and Education in Sensory Disabilities at Texas Tech University. She also serves as a certified orientation and mobility specialist for the Texas Department of Assistive and Rehabilitative Services. Ms. Page has been employed as a certified orientation and mobility specialist for many years and has worked with diverse students in education and rehabilitation systems.

Rona Pogrund, Ph.D., is Professor, Special Education Program, College of Education, and coordinator of the program for teachers of students with visual impairments, at the Virginia Murray Sowell Center for Research and Education in Sensory Disabilities at Texas Tech University. She is the co-author of *TAPS: Teaching Age-Appropriate Purposeful Skills: An Orientation & Mobility Curriculum for Students with Visual Impairments* and co-editor of *Early Focus:*

Working with Young Children Who Are Blind or Visually Impaired and Their Families. Dr. Pogrund has published numerous journal articles and book chapters on the topics of service delivery and orientation and mobility for students with visual impairments.

Huan Zhang, B.A., is the founder, chief instructor, and executive director of Huan's Tai Chi in Cambridge, Massachusetts, as well as exercise instructor for the Helping Elders Living with Pain (HELP) study at the University of Massachusetts, Boston. He has 30 years' experience in Tai Chi Ch'uan and other Chinese martial arts forms. Mr. Zhang is the author of *Seeing Beyond the Tai Chi Footprint: Sixteen Essential Principles* and has led lectures, seminars, and demonstrations on tai chi practice across the United States.

CONTRIBUTOR

John Clare, M.A., is a teacher of the blind and visually impaired and a certified orientation and mobility instructor based in Alaska. Recently retired from the Kenai Peninsula Borough School District, he is returning to his roots as a private contractor working with Alaska's rural visually impaired and blind population. Mr. Clare was awarded the O&M Citation of Excellence for Direct Service Award in 2002 from the Association for Education and Rehabilitation of the Blind and Visually Impaired and the John Hewitt Memorial Award from the Alaska Governor's Committee on Employment and Rehabilitation of People with Disabilities in 2003.

CHAPTER 1

Vision Loss and Older Adults
Considerations for the Orientation and Mobility Professional

*Nora Griffin-Shirley
and Laura Bozeman*

The aging of America is evident wherever you look. People are living and working longer than ever before. We do not bat an eyelash at television commercials that advertise pharmaceuticals for age-related diseases or an online dating service for older adults.

The visibility of older people is a reflection of this population's growing size. The number of people "aged 65 and over is projected to be 83.7 million by 2050, almost double its estimated population of 43.1 million in 2012" (Ortman, Velkoff, & Hogan, 2014, p. 1). In 2010 the life expectancy was 76.2 years for men and 81.0 years for women (National Center for Health Statistics, 2014, p. 82), and is expected to improve in the coming years (Ortman et al., 2014).

Forty-five percent of people 65 years and older reported they have excellent or very good health while 6.2% needed personal care assistance from January to March 2014 (Ward, Clarke, Freeman, & Schiller, 2015). These results shed a somewhat positive light on the health status of older Americans, with the majority of them caring for themselves.

However, a certain percentage of older adults will be diagnosed with conditions that lead to impaired vision. The incidence of visual impairments increases with age (Dillon, Gu, Hoffman, & Ko, 2010) as a result of eye conditions that are more likely to occur in older people. In fact, 30 percent of all persons who have visual impairments are over 65 years of age (Desai, Pratt, Lentzner, & Robinson, 2001). One out of six individuals aged 70 years or over has a visual impairment, and the number of people over 80 with visual impairments doubles compared with persons aged 70–79 years (Dillon et al., 2010).

Visual impairment has a significant impact on the lives of older individuals. The onset of vision loss compromises the ability to drive, interact with others, and accomplish daily chores. Given the higher incidence of vision loss among older adults than among younger age groups, medical and rehabilitation professionals, as well as family members and the general public, should familiarize themselves with targeted programs and services intended to improve quality of life, such as orientation and mobility (O&M) services. This chapter presents information on the demographics and trends among a diverse aging population with age-related vision loss, psychosocial factors related to vision loss, the adjustment process, the definition and benefits of O&M services, and how these services are provided to older adults with vision loss.

DEMOGRAPHICS AND TRENDS AMONG THE AGING POPULATION WITH VISION LOSS

Research to identify the number of people with vision loss is problematic as a result of varying definitions of visual functioning, differing assessments, the size of age or ethnic groupings, the original source of prevalence data, limitations of data-collection procedures, assumptions made by researchers of prevalence studies, and the use of continuous-function models (Horowitz, Brennan, & Reinhardt, 2005; Massof, 2002; Wall Emerson & De l'Aune, 2010). The variability of populations studied, access to eye care within those populations, and varying patterns of surgical practice are also limiting factors on research that seeks to identify the prevalence of visual impairment and blindness (Eye Diseases Prevalence Research Group, 2004).

The Eye Diseases Prevalence Research Group (2004) examined eight population-based studies conducted in the 1990s to determine two things: the number of individuals over the age of 40 with blindness or low vision, and the causes of blindness and low vision in those cases. Results showed that as the number of people over the age of 80 increases within a population, so does the prevalence of blindness and low vision. Age-related macular degeneration in Caucasians, open-angle glaucoma and cataracts in African-Americans, and glaucoma in Hispanics were the major causes of blindness. In 50 percent of the cases, regardless of ethnicity, cataracts were the main cause of low vision.

Upon interviewing 1,219 people over 45 years of age via telephone, Horowitz et al. (2005) found that 17 percent of their participants reported having a visual impairment. With advancing age, the incidence of visual impairment increased as follows:

- 14.4 percent of participants ages 45–54
- 14.7 percent of participants ages 55–64
- 16.7 percent of participants ages 65–75
- 26.5 percent of participants over 75

The researchers called for more eye care services such as refraction services; medical and surgical intervention; rehabilitation training, including O&M, for older people with visual impairments; and general care.

Of the older adults who become visually impaired, a subpopulation of individuals has a hearing impairment. An estimated 5 to 20 percent of people over 70 years old are affected with both visual and hearing impairments, a condition known as dual sensory impairment. By 2030, there will be between 3.5 and 14 million older people with dual sensory impairments in America (U.S. Census Bureau as cited in Brennan & Bally, 2007).

People of certain ethnic backgrounds have higher incidences of certain chronic illnesses, such as hypertension, heart disease, and diabetes. Vision problems are more prevalent in non-Hispanic black and Mexican-American individuals than in non-Hispanic white individuals. The Native American population has the highest incidence of disabling conditions of any minority group within the U.S. (Dillon et al., 2010).

Vision loss, as well as balance problems, is more common among people living in poverty as well (Dillon et al., 2010). The combination of vision loss and balance problems can lead to falls that may result in hospitalization and even death (Couturier, 2010). Specifically, a lack of stereopsis and binocular visual acuity increases the risk of hip fracture (Ivers, Norton, Cumming, Butler, & Campbell, 2000); a binocular visual acuity of less than 20/60 puts a person over 60 years of age at risk of a hip fracture, and 40 percent of hip fractures reported by participants in one study were a result of vision problems (Ivers et al., 2000). Declines in both mobility and mental status frequently occur after a hip fracture, especially as time passes after a hospital discharge (Bentler et al., 2009). With this situation in mind, older adults may have a fear of falling. This fear of falling can be lessened through a combination of O&M training and biannual eye tests (Alma, Groothoff, Melis-Dankers, Suurmeijer, & van der Mei, 2013; Bentler et al., 2009).

Although the exact incidence of visual impairment among older adults is unknown, the population of older Americans with visual impairments—including those with dual sensory impairments—is increasing. These individuals require, and benefit from, O&M services.

PSYCHOLOGICAL FACTORS RELATED TO AGING, VISION LOSS, AND THE ADJUSTMENT PROCESS

Visual impairment can cause functional disabilities (see Sidebar 1.1), including an increased likelihood of falls, resulting in longer hospital stays and more doctor visits, and a decrease in psychological well-being (Horowitz et al., 2005). Horowitz et al. identified the following risk factors associated with vision loss:

- advanced age
- ethnicity (other than Hispanic)
- poor health
- lack of informal supports, such as family members and friends

When older adults experience vision loss, their social interactions can be negatively affected. People with vision loss are less likely to socialize with friends and participate in community activities than their sighted peers (Brouwer, Sadlo, Winding, & Hanneman, 2008; Crews & Campbell, 2001). Direct family relationships can also be affected.

Using data from the 2006 and 2008 Behavioral Risk Factor Surveillance System, an ongoing telephone health survey conducted by the Centers for Disease Control and Prevention, Li et al. (2011) explored the relationship between having a single or multiple age-related eye diseases (ARED) and health-related quality of life (HRQOL). The study specifically targeted mental distress and physical impairments in people aged 65 and older. Those with more than one ARED were generally older than those with a single ARED, and also reported having more problems with visual and physical impairments.

When examining the ways older people adjust to vision loss, it is important to be aware of the general attitude of the sighted population toward blindness. Brennan, Horowitz, and Reinhardt (2004) conducted a telephone survey of 861 people over the age of 55, exploring their attitudes, knowledge, and fears concerning vision loss and aging. Participants demonstrated a limited knowledge of aging and vision loss and tended to fear blindness more than other disabling conditions (with the exception of mental illness), but

SIDEBAR 1.1

Effects of Vision Loss on Older Adults

Older adults with vision loss experience many of the following effects:

- increased incidence of falls
- longer hospital stays and doctor visits
- isolation due to a decreased likelihood of socialization with friends and participation in community activities
- an increase in feelings of depression, frustration, helplessness, and insecurity; loss of confidence; and reduced self-esteem leading to a decline in overall mental health
- fear of blindness
- compromised communication (for those with both vision and hearing loss)

Other factors that may negatively affect older people with vision loss include:

- lack of informal supports such as family members and friends
- negative stereotypes of people with visual impairments

Source: Adapted from Griffin-Shirley, N., & Welsh, R. L. (2010). Teaching orientation and mobility to older adults. In W. R. Wiener, R. L. Welsh, & B. B. Blasch (Eds.), *Foundations of orientation and mobility: Vol. II. Instructional strategies and practical applications* (3rd ed., pp. 286–311). New York: AFB Press.

---

reported a somewhat positive attitude toward loss of vision in later life. Predictors of a more positive attitude toward blindness included younger age, higher income and education, experience with a nonrelative with a visual impairment, and awareness of aging and vision loss. Interestingly, having vision loss was not a predictor of attitude. Brennan et al. (2004) mention that as people age they may adopt negative stereotypes of persons with visual impairments. To dispel negative stereotypes that may be held by older people, the general public and persons who are blind or visually impaired need to be educated about vision loss, as well as how people successfully cope with low vision. O&M specialists can help develop these educational programs.

Often, an older person who becomes visually impaired has experienced other losses throughout the course of his or her lifetime. The coping strategies used in response to the individual's vision loss tend to be the same strategies he or she used in the past to deal with crisis situations. Older adults with vision loss may be more inclined to passively accept the loss, especially as compared to younger individuals who become blind. This passivity may also make older individuals more reliant upon others for assistance, rather than learning and using new compensatory skills such as O&M (Brennan & Bally, 2007).

Feelings of "anxiety, anger, dependence, depression, fear, frustration, guilt, helplessness, insecurity, irritability, loss of confidence, insecurity, marginalized or diminished self-identity, reduced self-esteem, depression, withdrawal, dependence, and a diminished sense of well-being" are all common reactions to vision loss (Brennan & Bally, 2007, p. 286). These feelings can make older adults reticent to seek rehabilitation training or utilize newly acquired compensatory skills and adaptive equipment (Brouwer et al., 2008; Watson, 1996). On the other hand, vision rehabilitation has a positive effect on older adults with visual impairments, increasing positive adaptation to vision loss, decreasing feelings of helplessness, improving mental health, and proposing a less vision-specific fear of falling (Alma et al., 2013; Moore, Steinman, Giesen, & Frank, 2006). O'Donnell (2005) advocates for "rehabilitation and psychosocial intervention early in the process of vision loss to preserve a sense of well-being and prevent depression and dependence" (p. 200). O'Donnell also suggests that rehabilitation professionals maintain their relationships with older individuals, to help these patients cope with progressive loss of vision.

Many people turn to religion when faced with a crisis situation such as the onset of low vision or blindness. Spirituality helps some older people cope with vision loss and enhances their success in a vision rehabilitation program. Religious entities also provide support services, such as home repair, transportation, and religious texts in braille, to older people, including those who are blind or visually impaired (Brennan & Bally, 2007). This relationship may be one an O&M specialist can call upon to facilitate a variety of assistance or services. For example, an O&M specialist may help a client contact their church or temple to see if the congregation can help make physical adaptations to the individual's home, such as adding railings to stairs.

Depression negatively affects vision rehabilitation outcomes for patients with low vision (Crumbliss, 2012). For example, Grant, Seiple, and Szlyk (2011) measured the psychological well-being of 18 older adults with low vision and their adaptation to their vision loss at the beginning and end of their reading rehabilitation program. The results indicated that severe depression had a negative effect on the achievement of their reading rehabilitation goals.

However, after training, the participants' adaptation to vision loss improved. To increase the success of patients in reaching their goals, Crumbliss (2012) suggests rehabilitation workers undergo training on the effects of vision loss on the mental health of older adults.

Professional counseling (Boerner, Reinhardt, & Horowitz, 2006; Horowitz, Reinhardt, & Boerner, 2005) and support groups for older adults with vision loss, their sighted spouses, and family members help all parties cope with the psychological aspects of visual impairment (Orr & Rogers, 2006; Wolffe, 2010). A more positive outlook, greater satisfaction with life, the chance to learn new coping strategies, and engagement in social interactions are some benefits of involvement in peer support groups for older adults with vision loss (Orr & Rogers, 2006). Support groups also help families understand the feelings of older adults with vision loss, and learn when and how to provide assistance to them (Cimarolli, Sussman-Skalka, & Goodman, 2004; Orr & Rogers, 2006; Van Zandt, Van Zandt, & Wang, 1994). For example, older adults with vision loss, as well as their spouses, may have a fear of the individual with the visual impairment traveling independently. When these fears are shared in counseling sessions or with support groups, group members with O&M training who are independent travelers can share their successes and struggles. Such sharing can have a beneficial effect, giving motivation to those group members who have not yet received, or who are currently engaged in, an O&M program.

Orientation and mobility specialists can assist older adults with vision loss and their families to improve their psychological well-being. Suggestions for ways in which O&M specialists can do this are listed in Sidebar 1.2.

PSYCHOLOGICAL IMPACT OF DUAL SENSORY IMPAIRMENT

Older people who are faced with both a visual and a hearing impairment may be confronted with additional challenges, such as the inability to communicate well with others; problems with mobility; other people's negative attitudes; and inadequate healthcare, residential, medical, and rehabilitation services. If older people decide to retire early due to the onset of both hearing and vision losses, their income may be negatively affected (Brennan & Bally, 2007). These challenges can adversely affect the psychological status of individuals with dual sensory impairments. It is estimated that major depressive disorder affects 18 percent of persons with dual sensory impairment and

> **SIDEBAR 1.2**
>
> ## Improving Psychological and Physical Well-Being: Strategies for Older Adults with Vision Loss and Their Families
>
> Following are strategies that O&M specialists can use with older clients and their family members to help improve their psychological and physical well-being:
>
> - Provide O&M training focused on the immediate needs stated by the client.
> - Discuss the benefits of peer support groups for the sharing of fears, challenges, and successes with O&M training.
> - Listen to family members' ideas and feelings about their loved ones who are receiving O&M services.
> - Reinforce guiding skills clients have learned and suggest that they teach these skills to family members.
> - Refer clients and their families for counseling when necessary.
> - Work collaboratively with other professionals when providing services.
> - Encourage older clients to advocate for themselves in matters of accessibility (such as getting ramps installed in their homes) and services (such as receiving a low vision examination).
> - Acquaint clients and their family members with agencies that can help make their homes more accessible, provide transportation services, and the like.

12 percent of persons with a vision loss or a hearing loss (Lupsakko, Mantyjarvi, Kautiainen, & Sulkava, 2002). Individuals with dual sensory impairment also commonly report problems with memory, leading to confusion (Brennan & Bally, 2007).

Engaging in social interactions can also be difficult for persons with dual sensory impairment since communication is compromised. Crews and Campbell (2004) reported that individuals with dual sensory impairment were less likely to socialize with friends or go to restaurants, churches, and movies than those with a single or no sensory impairment. O&M specialists can assist adults with dual sensory impairment to find ways to travel to destinations where social interaction can occur.

THE EFFECTS OF CAREGIVING ON FAMILY MEMBERS

Family members and spouses usually provide support to individuals with vision loss, but giving this care can take its toll. For example, studies of a single sensory loss have demonstrated a negative effect on the emotional well-being of spouses (Brennan & Bally, 2007). It is common for family caregivers to be overprotective of the individual with vision loss, which can lead to further disability. Involvement in vision rehabilitation programs has been shown to be an effective way to increase family-life satisfaction and to improve the family's knowledge of how to help their loved one with a visual impairment (Horowitz et al., 1998).

Silva-Smith, Theune, and Spaid (2007) identified the primary people who support individuals with vision loss, the types of support provided, and the level of burden or strain felt as a result of caregiving. The primary caregivers were spouses or adult children. They carried out transportation, shopping, and administrative tasks such as writing and balancing checks, writing letters, and reading mail. These caregivers felt mild burden or strain but reported a fairly high level of self-esteem as a caregiver. Because O&M specialists are responsible for teaching older adults with vision loss how to use public transportation, it is imperative that they be familiar with the research in this area of caregiver responsibility (Silva-Smith et al., 2007) so they can act as a resource for older adults and their families in exploring transportation options that will lessen the amount of driving required of caregivers.

DEFINITIONS AND BENEFITS OF O&M SERVICES FOR OLDER ADULTS

Orientation and mobility is the profession that teaches concepts and travel skills to people who are blind or have low vision across the lifespan. *Orientation* is defined as knowing where you are and where you are going in relation to significant landmarks in the environment. *Mobility* is the ability to move safely and efficiently from one place to another through indoor and outdoor environments (Hill & Ponder, 1976). O&M services are available to children and adults of all ages. This book describes the training provided to older adults with visual impairments.

Benefits of O&M Instruction

Benefits of O&M instruction include safe and efficient travel across environments, being in tune with one's surroundings, and improved mental and physical health. Psychological benefits include enhanced self-esteem, confidence, feelings of well-being (Brouwer et al., 2008), and overall quality of life (Yeung, LaGrow, Towers, Alpass, & Stephens, 2011). The resulting freedom of travel also reduces stress (Kuyk et al., 2004). Physically, O&M training can improve balance, posture, endurance, gait, coordination, and alleviate deconditioning due to inactivity. Reduction in the incidence of falls can also be a result of environmental modifications and a walking program (Campbell et al., 2005). For older adults with vision loss, O&M instruction that provides familiarization with walking paths that they can continue to use for exercise can contribute to building strength and endurance, thus reducing the likelihood of falling.

Prior to O&M instruction, it is not uncommon for older adults with vision loss to become isolated and withdrawn. The individual may no longer go out with friends or family, shop, attend religious services, or engage in leisure activities (such as gardening or exercising). After receiving O&M training, however, these individuals have the strategies and skills to re-engage in their daily life. This increased involvement can improve the quality of their life (Griffin-Shirley & Welsh, 2010).

Studies of the Effectiveness of O&M Services

In a study mandated by Congress, *Vision Rehabilitation for Elderly Individuals with Low Vision or Blindness* (Agency for Healthcare Research and Quality, 2004), the Secretary of Health and Human Services reviewed evidence of the efficacy of vision rehabilitation services, including O&M services, provided to older adults with vision loss. The quality of existing studies was rated by criteria developed by the Agency for Healthcare Research and Quality. After conducting a literature search, only three articles were found that met the criteria: two studies (Engel, Welsh, & Lewis, 2000; Soong, Lovie-Kitchin, & Brown, 2001) and one systematic review (Virgili & Rubin, 2003). Due to the lack of standardized assessment tools to measure the outcomes of O&M training in the two studies, the authors of *Vision Rehabilitation for Elderly Individuals with Low Vision or Blindness* concluded that the effectiveness of O&M instruction was inconclusive. Similarly, the review by Virgili and Rubin (2003) did not provide any conclusive, evidence-based research concerning the efficacy of O&M training. Despite this lack of standardized O&M assessment tools, checklists, such as the O&M Checklist (Jacobson, 2013) and the Checklist of O&M Instructional Areas and Related Objectives (Knott, 2002), were developed by O&M specialists to measure the post-instructional progress of O&M skills of people with visual impairments.

Researchers suggest studies focused on O&M services for older adults are warranted. For example, Brouwer et al. (2008) discussed the paucity of research that demonstrates the cost and benefits of mobility training for older adults funded by the government in The Netherlands. Yeung et al. (2011) called for further investigation regarding the relationship between an individual's ability to get around and his or her quality of life. The use of an identification cane on the daily functioning of older adults with vision loss also needs exploration (Zijlstra et al., 2009). In conclusion, more research examining the efficacy of O&M services is needed to determine its effectiveness.

PROVISION OF O&M SERVICES FOR OLDER ADULTS WITH VISION LOSS

Typically, older adults with vision loss first consult an eye care professional such as an optometrist or ophthalmologist. Prompted by a referral from an optometrist or ophthalmologist, they may then seek specialized low vision services (Watson & Echt, 2010). Depending on the comprehensiveness of the low vision service provider, O&M instruction may be delivered through the low vision provider. The low vision provider may make a referral for vision rehabilitation services or send the individual directly to a private-contractor O&M specialist (Massof, 1995; Watson & Echt, 2010).

Agencies providing O&M services, in addition to other vision rehabilitation services, include adult rehabilitation facilities for people who are visually impaired, independent living centers that serve individuals with disabilities, low vision clinics, and Blind Rehabilitation Centers run by the U.S. Department of Veterans Affairs. Individual O&M specialists also contract with federal, state, and private agencies to serve older adults with vision loss in their own homes and communities (Griffin-Shirley & Welsh, 2010). The number of hours allocated by federal, state, and private agencies for O&M services varies and is dependent on many factors, such as the individual's needs, the recommendations of the rehabilitation team, the amount of money allocated for O&M services through an agency, access to O&M specialists, and the time the specialists have to spend in a certain geographic area.

Older adults with vision loss receive O&M services through center-based or community-based itinerant programs, or a combination of both. A center-based program offers a complete personal adjustment program for their clients, with O&M services being an integral part of the total program. A community-based itinerant program delivers O&M instruction to older people where they live (at home, in assisted living care, or at a nursing facility) (Griffin-Shirley & Welsh, 2010; Watson & Echt, 2010). In some cases, older adults are served by a center-based program and also receive outreach services in their homes.

O&M specialists are part of a rehabilitation team that includes a variety of professionals, depending on the needs of the client. It is important for O&M specialists to work collaboratively with other team members and to know when to consult another professional about their clients' needs. Sidebar 1.3 provides a description of a number of the possible team members and when they might need to be consulted. While collaboration is discussed throughout the book, the rehabilitation team is also addressed specifically in Chapter 7, and collaboration among team members is discussed in detail in Chapter 8.

TRANSPORTATION

Assisting with transportation needs is another important service provided by O&M specialists for their older clients. A wide variety of transportation services are available to older adults with visual impairments, including buses, subways, paratransit services, taxies, airplanes, trains, and personal automobiles. These services are often provided by area agencies on aging, metropolitan transit authorities, or private companies. Some transportation systems, such as paratransit and special buses, require the completion of an application process before an older adult with vision loss can become a rider. In addition, transportation authorities in larger communities offer travel training and O&M training for those using public transit. O&M specialists can be instrumental in helping older adults with vision loss access and use these services (Dodson-Burk, Park-Leach & Myers, 2010). More information concerning transportation options is provided in Chapters 3 and 4.

SUMMARY

The number of individuals with vision loss is increasing, with a higher incidence of visual impairment seen in those over 80 years of age. O&M training can ameliorate some of the negative effects of vision loss (such as loss of independence, depression, and an increased incidence of falls). O&M training benefits older people with vision loss in many ways, including the following:

SIDEBAR 1.3

Collaboration with Professionals on the Rehabilitation Team

James Scott Crawford

It is important for O&M specialists to work in tandem with related professionals such as physical therapists and physicians and to consult them when questions arise about a particular client that is outside the specialist's expertise. Techniques and strategies that may work perfectly with clients who have no other conditions besides visual impairment may cause pain or further injury for a client with additional disabilities or conditions or may cause the client to be unsafe. It is not always clear which professional to approach for a specific need. The following list describes some of the professionals who commonly work as part of a rehabilitation team for older adults with vision loss. (See Chapter 8 for strategies for effective collaboration.)

PHYSICIANS AND OFFICE STAFF

In addition to physicians, O&M specialists may need to collaborate with other primary care providers such as nurse practitioners and physician's assistants. As with any exercise program, older clients should check with their physicians before beginning O&M training. Physical activity limitations placed by physicians should be specific, well defined, and closely followed by O&M specialists. If there is any uncertainty about a given limitation, the specialist should contact the physician. Having the client present may improve understanding among all three parties (Griffin-Shirley & Welsh, 2010; Ponchillia & Ponchillia, 1996).

It is important to maintain information flow between clients and their physicians. For example, the increased physical activity involved in O&M training may create the need to adjust medications, requiring consultation with the physician. For instance, a client with diabetes will need to closely monitor his or her blood sugar levels when undertaking an O&M program, and his or her doctor may need to assist with adjusting medications appropriately. Similarly, increased activity and increased stress may change the way many medications affect clients, including, but not limited to, medications that control blood pressure, seizures, ocular pressure, blood thickness, sodium and potassium levels, and urine output, to name a few.

(continued)

SIDEBAR 1.3 (*continued*)

PHYSICAL THERAPISTS

Physical therapists are rehabilitation professionals who work to restore function and mobility, relieve pain, and prevent disability. Physical therapists tend to focus on building stamina, strength, and increasing range of motion (Griffin-Shirley & Welsh, 2010).

OCCUPATIONAL THERAPISTS

Occupational therapists focus on helping clients perform specific tasks related to their work or daily living requirements (Corn & Lusk, 2010; Ponchillia & Ponchillia, 1996). Some occupational therapists perform assessments and training tasks that are also within the purview of certified low vision therapists and certified vision rehabilitation therapists.

RECREATIONAL THERAPISTS

Recreational therapists direct and organize activities such as sports, dramatics, games, and arts and crafts to help clients develop interpersonal relationships, socialize effectively, and increase confidence in order to participate in group activities. Consultation can facilitate maximum benefit from both recreational therapy and O&M programs. (See Chapter 6 for more information on exercise for older adults with vision loss.)

AUDIOLOGISTS

Audiologists determine the type and severity of a hearing impairment. These specialists assist with hearing aid prescriptions and perform adjustments to hearing aids in order to maximize functional hearing. Normally, hearing aids are set to amplify sounds in the frequencies commonly used in speech and to reduce other frequencies. Often, the sounds used in O&M are intentionally blocked or dampened by this kind of hearing aid setting. Audiologists can change hearing aid settings to clarify the sounds of traffic and other ambient noises that facilitate travel but muddle conversation. (See Chapter 2 for more information.)

SPEECH-LANGUAGE PATHOLOGISTS

Speech-language pathologists work with individuals who have difficulties with speech and language and assist with communication issues. For older clients with speech issues, O&M specialists can consult with a speech-language pathologist to clarify the types of information the client needs to communicate about during travel. With that information, speech-language pathologists can prioritize training that relates to the client's travel goals (Corn & Lusk, 2010).

> **LOW VISION THERAPISTS**
>
> Low vision therapists usually are O&M specialists, teachers of students with visual impairments, or vision rehabilitation therapists who have received additional training in low vision and are certified by the Academy for the Certification of Vision Rehabilitation and Education Professionals (ACVREP). These professionals provide visual efficiency training to individuals with vision loss and train them how to use their optical devices (Corn & Lusk, 2010).
>
> **VISION REHABILITATION THERAPISTS**
>
> Vision rehabilitation therapists are professionals who instruct people with visual impairments in adaptive techniques for completion of activities of daily living. They may be certified by ACVREP (Corn & Lusk, 2010).

- supports the ability to live safely at home
- helps individuals become more independent travelers
- reduces the incidence of falls
- improves psychological well-being

O&M training is provided through center-based programs, community-based itinerant programs, or a combination of the two, and is delivered by highly qualified certified professionals, called O&M specialists. These professionals are key members of the rehabilitation teams that work with older adults and are instrumental in the identification of needs, development of rehabilitation goals, and successful implementation of instructional programs to meet those goals.

LEARNING ACTIVITIES

1. Interview a certified O&M specialist about his or her experiences providing training to older adults with vision loss. Ask the following questions:
    a. What are the challenges he or she faced?
    b. Which O&M techniques worked well with older adults?
    c. Which services were provided to family members of older adults when the specialist was teaching O&M skills?

2. Interview an older adult with vision loss. Find out the following information:

    a. how he or she was referred for O&M services

    b. the individual's feelings regarding the services he or she received

    c. his or her suggestions for O&M specialists when teaching older adults with vision loss

    d. his or her advice for other older adults who need O&M services

3. Visit a rehabilitation center for individuals with visual impairments and observe O&M lessons with older adults with vision loss. Write a 1–2 page summary of what occurred during the lessons and your reflections on the provision of O&M services to this population.

4. Reflect on your older family members.

    a. Has anyone experienced a vision loss?

    b. If so, how did your family cope with this family member?

    c. List the effective and ineffective coping strategies your family used.

References

Agency for Healthcare Research and Quality. (2004). *Vision rehabilitation for elderly individuals with low vision or blindness. Technology assessment.* Rockville, MD: U.S. Department of Health and Human Services. Retrieved from http://www.cms.gov/Medicare/Coverage/InfoExchange/downloads/rtcvisionrehab.pdf

Alma, M. A., Groothoff, J. W., Melis-Dankers, B. J. M., Suurmeijer, T. P. B. M., & van der Mei, S. F. (2013). The effectiveness of a multi-disciplinary group rehabilitation program on the psychosocial functioning of elderly people who are visually impaired. *Journal of Visual Impairment & Blindness, 107*(1), 5–16.

Bentler, S. E., Liu, L., Obrizan, M., Cook, E. A., Wright, K. B., Geweke, J. F., . . . Wolinsky, F. D. (2009). The aftermath of hip fracture: Discharge placement, functional status change, and mortality. *American Journal of Epidemiology, 170*(10), 1290–1299.

Boerner, K., Reinhardt, J. P., & Horowitz, A. (2006). The effect of rehabilitation service use on coping patterns over time among older adults with age-related vision loss. *Clinical Rehabilitation, 20*(6), 478–487.

Brennan, M., & Bally, S. J. (2007). Psychosocial adaptations to dual sensory loss in middle and late adulthood. *Trends in Amplification, 11*(4), 281–300.

Brennan, M., Horowitz, A., & Reinhardt, J. P. (2004). Understanding older Americans' attitudes, knowledge, and fears about vision loss and aging. *Journal of Social Work in Disability & Rehabilitation, 3*(3), 17–38.

Brouwer, D. M., Sadlo, G., Winding, K., & Hanneman, M. I. G. (2008). Limitations in mobility: Experiences of visually impaired older people. *British Journal of Occupational Therapy, 71*(10), 414–421.

Campbell, A. J., Robertson, M. C., LaGrow, S. J., Kerse, N. M., Sanderson, G. F., Jacobs, R. J., . . . Hale, L. A. (2005). Randomized controlled trial of prevention of falls in people aged ≥75 with severe visual impairment: The VIP trial. *The British Medical Journal, 331*, 817–820.

Cimarolli, V. R., Sussman-Skalka, C. J., & Goodman, C. R. (2004). "Program for partners": Support groups for partners of adults with visual impairments. *Journal of Visual Impairment & Blindness, 98*(2), 90–98.

Corn, A. L., & Lusk, K. E. (2010). Perspectives on low vision. In A. L. Corn & J. N. Erin (Eds.), *Foundations of low vision: Clinical and functional perspectives* (2nd ed., pp. 3–34). New York: AFB Press.

Couturier, J. A. (2010). Falling: Prevalence, risk factors, and interventions [Chapter appendix]. In W. R. Wiener, R. L. Welsh, & B. B. Blasch (Eds.), *Foundations of orientation and mobility: Vol. II. Instructional strategies and practical applications* (3rd ed., pp. 309–311). New York: AFB Press.

Crews, J. E., & Campbell, V. A. (2001). Health conditions, activity limitations, and participation restrictions among older people with visual impairments. *Journal of Visual Impairment & Blindness, 95*(8), 453–467.

Crews, J. E., & Campbell, V. A. (2004). Vision impairment and hearing loss among community-dwelling older Americans: Implications for health and functioning. *American Journal of Public Health, 94*(5), 823–829.

Crumbliss, K. (2012). Depression and vision rehabilitation: Recognizing and managing this prevalent co-morbidity. *Visibility: Education and Research from Envision, 6*(1), 1–5.

Desai, M., Pratt, L. A., Lentzner, H., & Robinson, K. N. (2001). *Trends in vision and hearing among older Americans* (Aging Trends No. 2). Hyattsville, MD: Centers for Disease Control and Prevention, National Center for Health Statistics.

Dillon, C. F., Gu, Q., Hoffman, H. J., & Ko, C. W. (2010). *Vision, hearing, balance, and sensory impairment in Americans aged 70 years and over: United States, 1999–2006* (NCHS Data Brief No. 31). Hyattsville, MD: Centers for Disease Control and Prevention, National Center for Health Statistics. Retrieved from http://www.cdc.gov/nchs/data/databriefs/db31.pdf

Dodson-Burk, B., Park-Leach, L., & Myers, L. (2010). Teaching the use of transportation systems for orientation and mobility. In W. R. Wiener, R. L. Welsh, & B. B. Blasch (Eds.), *Foundations of orientation and mobility: Vol. II. Instructional strategies and practical applications* (3rd ed., pp. 420–461). New York: AFB Press.

Engel, R. J., Welsh, R. L., & Lewis, L. J. (2000). Improving the well-being of vision-impaired older adults through orientation and mobility training and rehabilitation: An evaluation. *RE:view, 32*(2), 67–76.

Eye Diseases Prevalence Research Group. (2004). Causes and prevalence of visual impairment among adults in the United States. *Archives of Ophthalmology, 122*(4), 477–485.

Grant, P., Seiple, W., & Szlyk, J. P. (2011). Effect of depression on actual and perceived effects of reading rehabilitation for people with central vision loss. *Journal of Rehabilitation Research & Development, 48*(9), 1101–1108.

Griffin-Shirley, N., & Welsh, R. L. (2010). Teaching orientation and mobility to older adults. In W. R. Wiener, R. L. Welsh, & B. B. Blasch (Eds.), *Foundations of orientation and mobility: Vol. II. Instructional strategies and practical applications* (3rd ed., pp. 286–311). New York: AFB Press.

Hill, E., & Ponder, P. (1976). *Orientation and mobility techniques: A guide for the practitioner.* New York: American Foundation for the Blind.

Horowitz, A., Bird, B., Goodman, C. R., Flynn, M., Reinhardt, J. P., DeFini, J., . . . Silverstone, B. (1998). *Vision rehabilitation and family services: Maximizing functional and psychosocial status for both older visually impaired adults and their families* (Final report submitted to the AARP Andrus Foundation). New York: Lighthouse International, Arlene R. Gordon Research Institute.

Horowitz, A., Brennan, M., & Reinhardt, J. P. (2005). Prevalence and risk factors for self-reported visual impairment among middle-aged and older adults. *Research on Aging, 27*(3), 307–326.

Horowitz, A., Reinhardt, J. P., & Boerner, K. (2005). The effect of rehabilitation on depression among visually disabled older adults. *Aging & Mental Health, 9*(6), 563–570.

Ivers, R. Q., Norton, R., Cumming, R. G., Butler, M., & Campbell, A. J. (2000). Visual impairment and risk of hip fracture. *American Journal of Epidemiology, 152*(7), 633–639.

Jacobson, W. H. (2013). *The art and science of teaching orientation and mobility to persons with visual impairments* (2nd ed.). New York: AFB Press.

Knott, N. I. (2002). *Teaching orientation and mobility in the schools: An instructor's companion.* New York: AFB Press.

Kuyk, T., Elliott, J. L., Wesley, J., Scilley, K., McIntosh, E., Mitchell, S., & Owsley, C. (2004). Mobility function in older veterans improves after blind rehabilitation. *Journal of Rehabilitation Research & Development, 41*, 337–346.

Li, Y., Crews, J. E., Elam-Evans, L. D., Fan, A. Z., Zhang, X., Elliott, A. F., & Balluz, L. (2011). Visual impairment and health-related quality of life among elderly adults with age-related eye diseases. *Quality of Life Research, 20*(6), 845–852.

Lupsakko, T., Mantyjarvi, M., Kautiainen, H., & Sulkava, R. (2002). Combined hearing and visual impairment and depression in a population aged 75 years and older. *International Journal of Geriatric Psychiatry, 17*(9), 808–813.

Massof, R. W. (1995). A systems model for low vision rehabilitation. I. Basic concepts. *Optometry and Vision Science, 72*(10), 725–736.

Massof, R. W. (2002). A model of the prevalence and incidence of low vision and blindness among adults in the U.S. *Optometry and Vision Science, 79*(1), 31–38.

Moore, J. E., Steinman, B. A., Giesen, J. M., & Frank, J. J. (2006). Functional outcomes and consumer satisfaction in the independent living program for older individuals who are blind. *Journal of Visual Impairment & Blindness, 100*(5), 285–294.

National Center for Health Statistics. (2014). *Health, United States, 2013: With special feature on prescription drugs.* Hyattsville, MD: Centers for Disease Control and Prevention. Retrieved from http://www.cdc.gov/nchs/data/hus/hus13.pdf

O'Donnell, C. (2005). The greatest generation meets its greatest challenge: Vision loss and depression in older adults. *Journal of Visual Impairment & Blindness, 99*(4), 197–208.

Orr, A. L., & Rogers, P. (2006). *Aging and vision loss: A handbook for families.* New York: AFB Press.

Ortman, J. M., Velkoff, V. A., & Hogan, H. (2014). *An aging nation: The older population in the United States. Population estimates and projections* (P25-1140). Washington, DC: U.S. Department of Commerce, Economics and Statistics Administration, U.S. Census Bureau.

Ponchillia, P. E., & Ponchillia, S. V. (1996). *Foundations of rehabilitation teaching with persons who are blind or visually impaired.* New York: AFB Press.

Silva-Smith, A. L., Theune, T. W., & Spaid, P. E. (2007). Primary support persons for individuals who are visually impaired: Who they are and the support they provide. *Journal of Visual Impairment & Blindness, 101*(2), 113–118.

Soong, G. P., Lovie-Kitchin, J. E., & Brown, B. (2001). Does mobility performance of visually impaired adults improve immediately after orientation and mobility training? *Optometry and Vision Science, 78*(9), 657–666.

Van Zandt, P. L., Van Zandt, S. L., & Wang, A. (1994). The role of support groups in adjusting to visual impairment in old age. *Journal of Visual Impairment & Blindness, 88*(3), 244–252.

Virgili, G., & Rubin, G. (2003). Orientation and mobility training for adults with low vision. *Cochrane Database of Systematic Reviews, 4.*

Wall Emerson, R. S., & De l'Aune, W. R. (2010). Research and the orientation and mobility specialist. In W. R. Wiener, R. L. Welsh, & B. B. Blasch (Eds.), *Foundations of orientation and mobility: Vol. I. History and theory* (3rd ed., pp. 569–596). New York: AFB Press.

Ward, B. W., Clarke, T. C., Freeman, G., & Schiller J. S. (March, 2015). *Early release of selected estimates based on data from the January–September 2014 National Health Interview Survey.* Data Table for Figure 11.3. Percentage of persons of all ages who had excellent or very good health, by age group and sex: United States, January–September 2014 & Figure 12.1. Percentage of adults 65 and over who needed help. National Center for Health Statistics. Available from: http://www.cdc.gov/nchs/nhis.htm.

Watson, G. R. (1996). Older adults with low vision. In A. L. Corn & A. J. Koenig (Eds.), *Foundations of low vision: Clinical and functional perspectives* (pp. 363–394). New York: AFB Press.

Watson, G. R., & Echt, K. V. (2010). Aging and loss of vision. In A. L. Corn & J. N. Erin (Eds.), *Foundations of low vision: Clinical and functional perspectives* (2nd ed., pp. 871–916). New York: AFB Press.

Wolffe, K. E. (2010). Rehabilitation services for adults with low vision: Personal, social, and independent living needs. In A. L. Corn & J. N. Erin (Eds.), *Foundations of low vision: Clinical and functional perspectives* (2nd ed., pp. 729–759). New York: AFB Press.

Yeung, P., LaGrow, S., Towers, A., Alpass, F., & Stephens, C. (2011). The centrality of O&M in rehabilitation programs designed to enhance quality of life: A structural equation modelling analysis. *International Journal of Orientation & Mobility, 4*(1), 10–20.

Zijlstra, G. A., van Rens, G. H., Scherder, E. J., Brouwer, D. M., van der Velde, J., Verstraten, P. F., & Kempen, G. (2009). Effects and feasibility of a standardized orientation and mobility training in using an identification cane for older adults with low vision: Design of a randomized controlled trial. *BMC Health Services Research, 9*, 1–11.

CHAPTER 2

Sensory Changes with Age
Assessment Strategies for Older Adults with Visual Impairment

Laura Bozeman and Ken Bozeman

Adults in developed countries are living as much as 10 years longer than their parents did. This extended longevity can be attributed to better health that postpones complications typically associated with aging (Vaupel, 2010). This trend of living longer indicates that many older adults are able to recover from illness and injury or may be living longer with physical, mental, and sensory changes common to aging (Griffin-Shirley & Welsh, 2010).

Although some complications of aging may be experienced at a later age, these issues have not been eliminated altogether. Along with wear-and-tear disorders like osteoarthritis, older adults can experience a general decline in mental faculties, including the ability to quickly process and remember information. In addition, sensory changes that are a common result of advancing age may, if not identified and addressed, be mistaken for cognitive problems or the inability to live independently by families, caregivers, and related service professionals (Crews & Campbell, 2004; Riddering, 2008).

This chapter addresses sensory changes that occur with age and the impact on the need for orientation and mobility (O&M) services for the older adult with visual impairments. Particular attention is paid to the loss of hearing as another critical sense. Since vision and hearing are both distance senses, providing information about the environment not immediately adjacent to the individual, when one is diminished, the other plays a critical adaptive role (Sense, 2013). If a person with vision loss is also hearing impaired, the ability of the individual to use hearing to compensate for the visual impairment is reduced. The effects of aging on taste, smell, and touch are also considered.

Assessment strategies are presented for the O&M specialist to consider. A sample intake and assessment form is included as well.

AGING AND THE VISUAL SYSTEM

As the adult ages, many structures of the eye change as well. The cornea becomes less sensitive, so an injury may not be detected. The pupil decreases in size and may be slower to react to changes in lighting. These pupillary changes require more light and more transition time for the individual to perform given tasks. In addition, the lens becomes less flexible and less translucent, compromising focus at near. In general, visual acuity (sharpness of vision) and the ability to distinguish colors decrease with age (Faye, 1984). In addition to these typical age-related vision changes, there are disorders of the eye that become more common with aging, including cataracts, glaucoma, age-related macular degeneration, and diabetic retinopathy.

These changes and disorders have functional implications, including loss of visual acuity (cataracts) and/or restrictions in peripheral and central visual fields (glaucoma). Cortical or cerebral incidents (stroke) can also cause, or be the result of, age-related vision complications. Many of the changes resulting from age-related visual abilities as well as disorders are gradual and may not result in total blindness; however, the impact on the individual is often significant and may require services from an O&M specialist—a professional trained to teach the concepts and skills necessary for a person with a visual impairment to travel safely. O&M specialists serving the adult population note an increase in the proportion of older adults in their caseloads (Griffin-Shirley & Welsh, 2010).

Ocular Disorders Common to Older Adults

There are four eye conditions that are the most common causes of vision loss among older adults: cataracts, glaucoma, age-related macular degeneration (ARMD), and diabetic retinopathy. Stroke, although not a visual condition, can also have a significant effect on vision. Some of these diseases have an impact on visual acuity while others affect peripheral vision or the ability to process visual information (Colenbrander, 2009; Faye, 1984).

Cataracts

A cataract is the clouding of the normally clear lens within the eye that can eventually cause a reduction in visual acuity, the ability to determine detail, or simply result in blurred vision. Cataracts may cause increased difficulty with glare and the ability to distinguish color, and a reduction in contrast sensitivity, as well.

Once a cataract reaches a stage where it interferes with an individual's everyday life, it may be removed surgically. Surgical removal is usually a quick and safe solution. Often the surgeon is able to insert a synthetic intraocular lens implant to allow the eye to focus, usually at a distance (Fagerström, 1994).

There may be contraindications for surgery or for an intraocular lens implant. In these cases, O&M instruction may be required to teach an older adult with cataracts to use other senses to support orientation and safe travel.

Glaucoma

While vision loss due to glaucoma can occur suddenly, it usually occurs so painlessly and gradually that glaucoma is sometimes called the "silent thief of sight." Often, an individual is not aware of the loss until a considerable amount of functional vision has been lost (Faye, 1984). With glaucoma, the overproduction of a fluid in the eye, called the aqueous, or failure of the aqueous to drain properly, causes pressure within the globe that can eventually damage the optic nerve. Routine intraocular pressure checks, as well as comprehensive dilated eye exams to look at the back of the eye, are crucial for older adults because they can detect subtle changes of the optic nerve in patients without any visual symptoms. Usually, peripheral vision is the first to be affected in glaucomatous vision loss. If left untreated, tunnel vision may occur, followed by impairment to central vision (Faye, 1984). Glaucoma is a chronic condition that must be monitored for life. Often, glaucoma can be effectively treated with medications that hold the progress of the disease at bay, and with proper monitoring and treatment, can be managed to minimize limitations to vision or lifestyle. For this reason, early detection is critical.

An older adult's mobility can be affected at the initial onset of glaucoma (peripheral field loss) and with the progression of the disease. A loss in the peripheral field can limit an individual's ability to travel safely without a mobility device. Peripheral vision warns the individual of drop-offs, furniture, and other obstacles that could cause him or her to trip or fall. O&M instruction is beneficial in such circumstances to teach the best use of remaining vision, as well as how other senses support safe travel.

Age-Related Macular Degeneration

ARMD is the most common eye disorder in adults 60 years of age and older. Research studies report that 30 percent of older adults have some form of ARMD. ARMD has two forms. The more common dry form manifests as a gradual, progressive loss of the ability to determine details, a decrease in contrast sensitivity, and eventually, a loss of the ability to identify colors due to the deterioration of the macula, the most sensitive part of the retina for sharp central vision. The older adult with ARMD may have difficulty reading street signs and text, recognizing faces, and performing any task that requires attention to, or awareness of, visual detail. The less common wet form of ARMD progresses more quickly than the dry form. It involves the deterioration of the macula with the addition of intraocular bleeding (Faye, 1984).

A client with ARMD will not become blind as a result of the disease since ARMD leaves peripheral vision intact (Mogk & Mogk, 2003). O&M specialists teach older adults with ARMD to use their remaining vision, low vision aids, and other sensory information to support effective orientation and safe travel.

Diabetic Retinopathy

Vision loss from diabetes, known as diabetic retinopathy, occurs when the disease weakens the blood vessels in the retina, causing blind spots and blurred vision. The development of diabetic retinopathy is linked to the amount of time an individual has had the disease. In the beginning stages, the blood vessels may rupture and bleed, causing problems with central vision. If left untreated, the progression can cause the retina to detach and may result in permanent vision loss. For the older adult with diabetes, visual abilities can fluctuate—even during a given day—which can lead to feelings of frustration and insecurity (Faye, 1984).

The main treatments for diabetic retinopathy are laser photocoagulation and vitrectomy. Laser photocoagulation therapy can stop the blood vessels from leaking by sealing the source of the bleeding. In some cases, a vitrectomy—a procedure in which the normally clear vitreous fluid of the eye, which is now compromised due to the bleeding, is removed and replaced with a clear liquid—may be needed (Faye, 1984).

People with diabetic retinopathy can benefit from O&M instruction. Since diabetes affects the entire body, the O&M specialist working with a diabetic individual must be aware of any neuropathy (lack of feeling in the extremities) that may make it difficult for a client to discern and use tactile information (Milligan, 1998). Implications for O&M include difficulty detecting inclines, declines, surface changes, and drop-offs. Also, blisters, cuts, and other forms of injury may go unnoticed due to neuropathy and take extended time to heal. People with diabetes must also monitor the insulin they take to regulate their blood sugar level in accordance with the increased exercise required during O&M lessons. Insulin regulation is critical to a diabetic client's stamina, ability to attend to the lesson, and general well-being. Due to changes in blood sugar levels and the balance of food intake, the time of day for the lesson is also important for the O&M specialist to consider (Griffin-Shirley & Welsh, 2010; Rosen & Crawford, 2010).

Neurological Considerations for Vision Loss in the Older Adult

Stroke is included here since it occurs more frequently in older adults. A stroke may occur from a blockage and restricted blood flow to the brain or a hemorrhage and bleeding in the brain, particularly on the right side (Colenbrander, 2009). Treatment depends on the site and seriousness of the injury. Strokes may result in vision-related problems such as nystagmus and field deficits (right and left hemianopsia) (Warren, 2008). Frequently, homonymous hemianopsias occur and can have a negative impact on mobility (Kerkhoff, 2000).

O&M instruction can be very helpful for the older adult as part of rehabilitation for a stroke. In addition to visual concerns, the client may have unilateral weakness, speech difficulties, or both, residual to the stroke. Thus, the older adult recovering from a stroke usually has many professionals assisting with recovery. In addition to medical personnel, occupational therapists, physical therapists, audiologists, and speech-language pathologists are examples of related service professionals involved in the rehabilitation process. Teamwork is paramount for the rehabilitation to be integrative and effective.

Charles Bonnet Syndrome

A condition called Charles Bonnet Syndrome does not easily fit into the common categories of eye conditions, but does warrant discussion. First described by Charles Bonnet in the 1700s, it is the occurrence of complex visual hallucinations in people with vision loss (Vukicevic & Fitzmaurice, 2008). Charles Bonnet Syndrome can occur at any age, but is more common in older adults with vision loss. Charles Bonnet Syndrome can be described as the brain's reaction to visual impairment. Similar to phantom limb syndrome, it is thought to be a type of misfire in the brain. The images in the hallucination often appear smaller in scale than the physical surroundings and occur in otherwise mentally healthy individuals. There is no prescribed treatment that consistently improves the condition, though it is helpful if the individual realizes the hallucinations are visual and not mental (Orr & Rogers, 2006).

The main concern with Charles Bonnet Syndrome is that the older adult, as well as his or her family and friends, may mistakenly attribute the hallucinations to mental illness or dementia. For this reason, researchers fear that the condition is vastly underreported (Vukicevic & Fitzmaurice, 2008). It usually subsides after 12 to 18 months, once the brain is accustomed to the vision loss (Griffin-Shirley & Welsh, 2010; Orr & Rogers, 2006).

The older adult with Charles Bonnet Syndrome may be unsure if the images he or she sees are real or hallucinations. This confusion can have an impact on O&M instruction while the client attempts to sort out real and meaningful clues and landmarks. There is some comfort in knowing that the condition is not permanent (Orr & Rogers, 2006).

AGING AND THE AUDITORY SYSTEM

The older adult with vision loss typically depends on his or her sense of hearing for environmental information and orientation clues. It is therefore important for the O&M specialist to understand the impact of any hearing loss a client may be experiencing. To understand an audiogram or narrative report about an older client's hearing, the O&M specialist must first know a little about how hearing works and the hearing disorders common to the older adult. The O&M specialist can then have a better idea of the functional implications of a hearing loss for the older client with a visual impairment and the possible impact this loss may have on travel.

How Hearing Works

As sound enters the ear canal, it travels toward the eardrum (or tympanic membrane). (See Figure 2.1 for a diagram of the ear.) When the sound strikes the eardrum, it causes a vibration similar to that of the head of a drum when struck by a drumstick. The vibrations of the eardrum in turn set the bones of the middle ear (called the ossicles) in motion. The ossicles are responsible for transmitting sound from the eardrum to the cochlea. The cochlea is a snail-shaped structure that contains the fluids of the inner ear and hair cells that, when stimulated, send the auditory signal to the brain. With each vibration, the ossicles press into the oval window in the cochlea, thus creating a hydraulic wave within the cochlea. It is this wave that moves the hair cells, creating the sensation of sound.

Types of Hearing Loss

There are two main categories of hearing loss, *conductive* and *sensorineural*. Each type refers to the anatomical area affected, and each has its own challenges in treatment and rehabilitation (Lawson & Wiener, 2010). It is possible to have a loss that combines both conductive and sensorineural elements. The functional implications of a mixed loss will vary depending on the severity of each component.

Conductive Hearing Loss

Conductive hearing loss relates to problems in the transmission or conduction of the sound wave from the external ear (called the pinna) to the oval

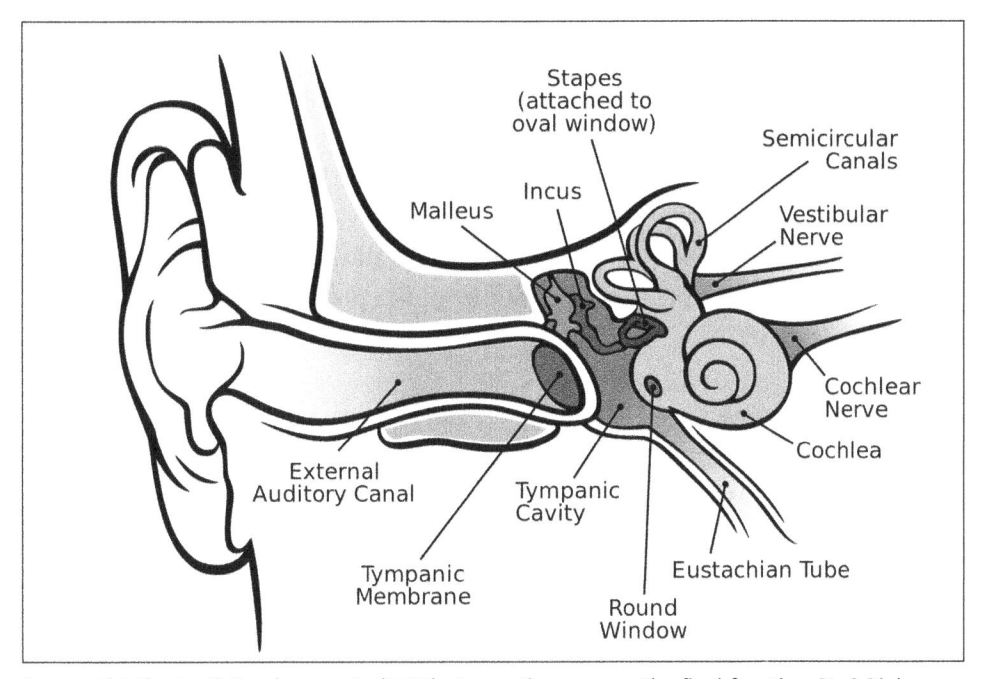

Source: Chittka, L., & Brockmann, A. (2005). Perception space—The final frontier. *PLoS Biology,* 3(4), e137.

FIGURE **2.1**

Diagram of the Human Ear

The stylized image shows the parts of the inner ear including the malleus, incus, stapes (attached to oval window), semicircular canals, vestibular nerve, cochlear nerve, cochlea, eustachian tube, round window, tympanic cavity, tympanic membrane, and external auditory canal.

window of the cochlea. A blockage in the ear canal, perforation of the eardrum, fracture of one of the bones or ossicles, or the presence of fluid in the middle ear are all examples of impairments that impede the conduction of the sound signal to the fluids of the inner ear. Conductive hearing loss may make conversation and environmental sounds seem muffled. If these sounds are amplified, competing noise is filtered out and the older adult may be able to use them for social interaction or safe travel (Lawson & Wiener, 2010). While the hearing loss resulting from conductive causes is usually temporary, the O&M specialist should be aware that conductive losses can have an impact on the older client's ability to correctly interpret sound clues. Many of these causes of conductive hearing loss are treatable with proper medication or surgical intervention.

Functionally, conductive hearing loss that causes a blockage in the outer or middle ear can make an individual's voice sound louder than normal to him- or herself. (It is possible to simulate this condition by covering the ears tightly with both hands and speaking. The result will be a louder and more hollow-sounding quality of the voice.) An older adult with this type of blockage may speak at a lower volume than normal, which may lead to a variety of O&M considerations. For example, an older adult who is speaking at a low volume may have trouble soliciting aid from the public as he or she may have difficulty being heard.

Sensorineural Loss

Sensorineural hearing loss refers to a disruption of the sound at the cochlea or beyond and is usually permanent. Sensorineural hearing loss is frequently caused by damage to the hair cells within the cochlea due to aging (called presbycusis) and overexposure to loud noise. In addition, sensorineural loss can be caused by tumors on the auditory nerve (the eighth cranial nerve), viral or bacterial infections of the inner ear, and ototoxins, pharmaceuticals that can cause hearing damage, such as aspirin and some mycin drugs (DiSogra & Weir, 1993).

A sensorineural loss may cause a client to speak at a higher volume than usual. The older adult with sensorineural loss may have an impaired ability to understand speech in noisier environments, which can affect not only communication and socialization, but the ability to understand instructions from the O&M specialist. Information from environmental sounds will, most likely, be diminished in clients with sensorineural hearing loss. The usual treatment for sensorineural hearing loss involves amplification in the form of hearing aids.

Central Auditory Processing Disorders

Central auditory processing disorder is a condition that affects understanding separately from a sensory hearing loss. As age increases, the incidence of auditory processing problems increases as well (Dillon, 2001). Central auditory processing refers to the efficiency and effectiveness by which the central nervous system utilizes auditory information. A central auditory processing disorder, then, refers to difficulties in the perceptual processing of auditory information in the central nervous system (Working Group on Auditory Processing Disorders, 2005). Common complaints from patients with auditory processing issues are difficulty hearing in background noise, difficulty following directions, needing to ask for repetition, and difficulty with localization (Dillon, 2001; Shinn, 2012).

Teaching clients with central auditory processing disorders may be difficult, as most hearing issues related to a central auditory processing disorder are subtle and can be interpreted as actual hearing loss. Traditional treatment, such as hearing aids, may not help and could make the situation worse. An older adult who has been treated for hearing loss but still has difficulties with environmental or speech signals should have further evaluation by an audiologist. For the older adult with vision loss, failure to process in any of these critical areas would have a direct effect on O&M instruction, including whether the client can accurately respond to traffic sounds, correctly interpret instructions, or respond to information from others.

Localization

Hearing loss can affect one of the more complex abilities of the human auditory system—the accurate pinpointing, or *localization,* of a sound source. Humans are not born with this skill, but rather learn it over time. An important component of localization is known as the *interaural time difference* (ITD; Dillon, 2001). The human ear is capable of detecting very small differences in the time and intensity of sounds. ITD relates to the time a given sound arrives at each ear. If a sound occurs directly in front of an individual, the resulting sound wave arrives at both ears at the same time. A sound that occurs to an individual's right side would arrive at the right ear first and at the left ear slightly later. This split-second difference gives the experienced listener cues about the location of the sound source. People with visual impairments use ITD-based localization in a variety of important ways, including determining the direction of traffic, identifying the presence of pedestrians, and sensing and interpreting environmental clues. Hearing loss can affect the ability to localize sound, especially when one ear is more impaired than the other ear (Lawson & Wiener, 2010).

Hearing Aids

One description of a hearing aid is that it "is basically a miniature public address system" (Dillon, 2001, p. 10). A hearing aid has a microphone to convert sound into electricity, an amplifier to increase the strength of the signal, a small receiver or loudspeaker to convert the electrical signal back into sound, and a battery to provide power.

Hearing aids can be a good option for the older adult with hearing loss. However, unlike eyeglasses, which can provide an immediate improvement in vision, hearing aids require instruction for effective use, and it can take time for clients to adjust to the devices (Dillon, 2001). Hearing aids are designed to maintain a set volume for different types of sounds, which can negate the information necessary for accurate localization. Recent advances allow the hearing aids used in an individual's right and left ears to communicate with one another wirelessly. This technology is a critical advancement for orientation and the client with hearing loss, as it can preserve some degree of localization and spatial awareness (see Sidebar 2.1).

It is important to make sure that older clients who have been prescribed hearing aids are wearing the aids and that the aids are in working order during O&M training. It is recommended that the O&M specialist learn how hearing aids work and how to perform basic troubleshooting for malfunctioning hearing aids. (For more information, see Troubleshooting Faulty Hearing Aids in Dillon, 2001, p. 111.)

If the O&M specialist suspects a malfunctioning hearing aid, the specialist should check the device. If the hearing aid is on and held in the cupped hand, it should generate feedback, making a squealing noise. If cupping the device does not cause squealing feedback, make sure the device is turned on. If it is turned on, check that the battery is installed correctly. Modern hearing aids signal when a battery is near depletion, but older wearers sometimes miss this signal and may not realize that a battery has died.

The hearing aid can be reset by opening and closing the battery door. This sets the program to default settings, which is most likely the correct program for the older adult. Any visible wax on the device should be removed with a tissue so it does not clog the aid.

SIDEBAR 2.1

> ### Bob: A Case Study in the Efficacy of Wireless Hearing Aids for Older Adults with Dual Sensory Impairment
>
> Bob is a 63-year-old man who has been blind since age 14. Bob had a successful career and traveled globally and independently with a dog guide. In his late 50s, Bob was diagnosed with Ménière's disease, which caused moderate hearing loss, tinnitus (ringing in the ears), and episodic vertigo (acute episodes of dizziness). Bob's ability to remain oriented in the environment was almost solely based on his ability to hear environmental cues. His hearing loss limited his ability to hear changes in the width of hallways and openings, to identify social cues, and to participate in conversations.
>
> Subsequent treatment adequately controlled the vertigo and tinnitus, but Bob still experienced a substantial hearing loss. He was fitted with digital hearing aids, but his orientation did not improve, nor did his ability to move through the environment effectively. Bob decided to retire because his orientation skills were so impaired by his hearing loss.
>
> Bob was eventually fitted with a new generation of hearing aids. His new pair of hearing aids communicated wirelessly with each other to more effectively preserve spatial awareness. These new hearing aids helped Bob regain his ability to hear traffic movement in a more functional way. He also demonstrated better orientation with the new aids, and was able to navigate indoors using auditory cues. After approximately one year with the new hearing aids, Bob's answers to the Abbreviated Profile of Hearing Aid Benefit questionnaire, a standardized self-reporting tool of hearing aid performance in a variety of environmental situations (Johnson, Cox, & Alexander, 2010), supported his improvement. Comparative measurements of orientation and mobility errors (Geruschat & De l'Aune, 1989) showed a decrease with the wireless technology (Bozeman & Bozeman, n.d.).
>
> Bob's experience suggests that improved technology in hearing aids holds promise to assist in localization for older adults with both visual and hearing loss.

Hearing aids are primarily designed to aid in understanding speech, which occurs in the frequency range of 500 to 4,000 Hertz (Hz). While conversation is important for socialization, for soliciting aid, and for knowing the location of pedestrians, the environmental sounds used for auditory orientation can occur outside of this "speech" range. Technological advances have improved the range and frequency-specific amplification required by the user. Hearing aids today are capable of processing a much broader range of 250 to 10,000 Hz, which includes many environmental sounds (Lawson & Wiener, 2010). Currently available hearing aids are usually digital and offer a higher degree of control and specificity to the amplified signal, which allows for a more accurate correction for an individual's hearing loss.

Some older clients will not be able to afford the most technologically advanced hearing aids, which can be quite expensive and are not covered by Medicare. For the older adult who has no other means of amplification, an alternative called a *personal sound amplifying product* (such as the Pocket Talker) may be a workable solution. Devices such as this are usually available at retail electronics stores. This is a relatively low-tech personal amplification option that increases the volume of the sounds in the area closest to the user. The device may help the older client with TV programs and close conversation, but does not have the features of a regular hearing aid and would not be effective for most outdoor travel. O&M instruction may be unsuccessful if hearing loss is not properly evaluated and treated. The O&M specialist should watch for any signs that an older adult may have a hearing loss and refer the client to an audiologist for assessment.

AGING AND THE SENSES OF SMELL AND TASTE

The sense of smell is often taken for granted until it diminishes. As with other senses, the ability to smell as well as distinguish between smells decreases with age (Boyce & Shone, 2006). Olfactory abilities decrease appreciably during the seventh decade and deterioration of taste abilities occurs concurrently. For the older adult, smell and taste are linked to the appeal of food and, ultimately, good nutrition, which is critical for the maintenance of health and strength.

Many theories of the causes of smell disorders revolve around sensory cell loss in the olfactory mucosa and a general loss of cognitive processing ability, especially for people in their 70s and beyond. The majority of taste disorders are actually a result of a decrease in the ability to smell (Boyce & Shone, 2006). In addition, the number of taste buds present on the tongue decreases with age.

The functional implications of smell disorders range from loss of enrichment (such as the inability to enjoy wonderful food aromas) to safety concerns (such as an inability to detect a natural gas leak or the presence of noxious fumes). The senses of smell and taste are linked, with most of the ability to taste coming from the sense of smell. The loss of smell (and taste) can result in decreased appetite, weight loss, and an overuse of condiments and seasonings (such as salt), which may be contraindicated due to hypertension or other health issues. For older adults with vision loss, a decreased ability to smell and taste may cause difficulties with the identification of foods.

For O&M instruction, smells act as clues about the older adult's surroundings. For example, the smell of popcorn may indicate proximity to a movie theater, and the smell of fresh bread may indicate that a bakery is nearby. These clues and cues provide rich environmental information and are helpful to orientation, especially when combined with information from other senses (Koutsoklenis & Papadopoulos, 2011).

AGING AND THE TACTILE SYSTEM

The sense of touch provides information about temperature, pain, and pressure. With age, tactile sensations may decrease due to poor diet or reduced blood flow. Changes in the tactile system are also safety concerns. Inaccurately detecting temperature can have an impact on choosing appropriate clothing or determining the temperature of foods or bath water. Decreased functioning of pain receptors may mask injuries. For the O&M client with a visual impairment, reduced tactile sensation can cause difficulty when distinguishing among objects in the environment as well as detecting drop-offs, declines, and inclines, and can limit the amount of information the client is able to perceive through the cane (Milligan, 1998).

An age-related decrease in tactile function may be exacerbated by peripheral neuropathy. Neuropathy indicates nerve damage and is a symptom or result of other ailments such as diabetes and kidney disorders. A side effect of neuropathy is the inability to feel pain, which can result in foot and leg ulcers that take a long time to heal (Ponchillia, 1993). Any change in tactile function can create complications for O&M instruction.

ADULT ASSESSMENT STRATEGIES

For the O&M specialist, assessment is a continuous process. There is value in initial, formal assessments as well as ongoing, informal assessments that take place as training evolves. Using the client's personal goals as a guide, the O&M specialist can develop an integrated plan that is individualized to the older adult with a visual impairment. The initial intake and functional assessment help inform that process.

Assessment

The best assessment processes take the whole client into account. For the older adult, background information, current health and medications, current vision and eye status, sensory abilities, any prior O&M skills, other disabilities, as well as conceptual knowledge and cognitive functioning, should all be considered. When performing an assessment, the goal of the O&M specialist is to discover all the abilities that the older adult brings to the training situation. Reports from other members of the rehabilitation team add to the picture of the older client. Figure 2.2 presents a sample form that can be used to guide and organize initial intake and assessment information.

The O&M assessment consists of two parts: the background assessment and the functional assessment. The background (or intake) assessment collects information, as self-reported by the client, and clinical results that then drive the functional assessment. The intake or background is important because the information collected provides a comprehensive depiction of the older adult, from his or her overall medical status, to family and friend supports, to previous O&M instruction and desires for the future. In the functional assessment, the instructor may review the client's ability to demonstrate the O&M skills that were reported as previously learned. It is best for the O&M specialist to perform the functional assessment in a variety of environments and to directly observe a client's functional abilities rather than rely solely on self-reporting or background information to determine the level of generalization and concept application used by the client. The O&M specialist can expand the categories listed in Figure 2.2 as needed to individualize the assessment for each client.

Intake

Background and Health. This category summarizes basic information about the client such as name, age, and referral source. This is also where the O&M specialist can engage the older adult and ask about his or her living situation and supports.

The eye report from the client's eye care specialist should be summarized to include clinical results such as diagnosis, visual acuity, and measures of visual fields. Other pertinent ocular information should be noted, such as whether any low vision devices have been prescribed. Clients should be asked to describe how they see in order to learn what they know about their visual condition and to give them the opportunity to describe their functional vision in their own words.

Intake and Functional Assessment Checklist

INTAKE (BASED ON OLDER ADULT'S SELF-REPORT)

Background and Health

Basic Details

Name: _____ Age: _____

Medical Dr. _____ Phone: _____

Referral source: _____

Living situation: _____

Supports (family/friends): _____

Information about Vision

Eye condition: _____

Visual acuity: _____

Peripheral fields: _____

Eye doctor: _____ Phone: _____

Date of last exam: _____ Prognosis: _____

Low vision exam: _____ Dr. _____

Current low vision devices: _____

Client's description of vision: _____

_____

Overall Health

General statement of health: _____

_____

☐ Additional health considerations
  ☐ Hearing loss
  ☐ Orthopedic
  ☐ Neurological issues
  ☐ Seizures
  ☐ Heart condition
  ☐ Respiratory
  ☐ Circulatory
  ☐ Other (specify): _____
☐ Functional complications
  ☐ Balance issues
  ☐ Stamina issues
  ☐ Memory issues
  ☐ Other (specify): _____

(continued)

FIGURE **2.2**

Sample Intake and Functional Assessment Checklist

☐ Medications (particularly those with side effects such as decreased vision, drowsiness, weakness, instability, etc.)
_____

Falls: Y   N   # in past 6 months: _____ Circumstances: _____

Functional Vision
Client description of vision:_____
_____
Functional vision observations during intake: _____
_____

Previous O&M Instruction: _____
_____

Previous Travel Routines: _____
_____

Present mobility indoors (self-report): _____
_____

Present mobility outdoors (self-report): _____
_____

Description of neighborhood: _____
_____

Transportation/Paratransit resources:_____
_____

Leisure Activities/Hobbies: _____
_____

Daily level of activity: _____
_____

Goals
Client's goals (including stated immediate need): _____
_____

Family's goals: _____
_____

Current Equipment
  ☐ Cane (if cane, include type, material, length, grip, tip, condition): _____
  ☐ Dog guide
  ☐ Electronic travel aids
  ☐ Caps, visors
  ☐ Sunglasses

FIGURE **2.2** *(continued)*

FUNCTIONAL ASSESSMENT
(BASED ON THE DESIRES/GOALS STATED BY THE OLDER ADULT)

Home Environment (Activities of daily living, routes to bathroom, dining area, living areas): _____
_____
_____

Residential Environment (Attend church, visit friends, go to the store):
_____
_____

Semi-Business Environment (Public transportation, alternate means of transportation, routes to community leisure): _____
_____
_____

Business Environment (Urban travel, more complicated routes, crowded, visually complex): _____
_____

All Environments (Personal safety, backup plans, alternate routes): _____
_____
_____

Environmental Considerations:
Lighting
    Increase: _____
    Decrease: _____
    Problem (glare): _____
    Transition (bright to dim; dim to bright): _____

Contrast
    Increase: _____
    Decrease: _____
    Color: _____
    Figure-ground (visual clutter): _____

Size
    Increase: _____
    Decrease: _____

Source: Adapted from work by Robert McCulley, MEd, Director, Northeast Regional Center for Vision Education, Institute for Community Inclusion, University of Massachusetts Boston.

Are there physical conditions that might have an impact on the older adult's movement, stamina, balance, or comfort during instruction? Arthritis is a common joint problem that occurs with age and can cause pain and stiffness that can influence the style and duration of the O&M lesson. Does the older client have medical conditions or prescribed medications that cause dizziness, seizures, or memory or balance issues?

Another part of the picture is the client's overall health. Is there an optimal time of day to schedule the lesson given medication concerns, insulin administration, or overall stiffness? Is there a diagnosed hearing loss?

Since the likelihood of falling increases with age (Fuller, 2000), noting if there were falls and the circumstances under which they occurred is good information to consider in O&M program planning. For older adults with a history of falls, incorporating other members of the team (such as occupational or physical therapists) will also benefit the O&M plan. More information about fall prevention is presented in Chapter 6.

Functional Vision Observations. The background report should contain a functional vision assessment if the older adult has received past vision services. The O&M specialist observes how the older adult functions during the intake and notes any difficulties with glare or lighting transitions and the need for increased contrast or size considerations.

Previous O&M Instruction and Travel Routines. If previous O&M instruction was provided, the older adult can discuss that instruction and how it was integrated into his or her daily routine. The O&M specialist should discuss any previous O&M instruction and compare the client's report to reports received from other instructors. Note the environments and skills that were introduced and the progress that was achieved. The older adult can relay his or her confidence in traveling in different environments and what transportation resources he or she used.

To begin to understand the client's current abilities and needs, the instructor can try to determine the older adult's travel routines, level of activity, leisure interests, hobbies, and motivation for instruction. This information can help establish a baseline and shape the individualized O&M program to reflect the interests of the older adult.

Goals. The assessment is based on the aspirations and desires of the older client with a visual impairment. What are the client's goals and what does he or she see as the most immediate need? What are the client's family members' goals for him or her? How these perceptions intersect is critical to the success of O&M instruction.

Current Equipment. Record any mobility devices currently used by the older adult such as a dog guide or electronic travel aids. If the client uses a long cane, include the type, material, length, grip, tip, and condition. Also note any other items such as sunglasses or caps or visors used by the client.

Functional Assessment

This portion of the O&M assessment provides the older adult with an opportunity to demonstrate his or her abilities and previous O&M training across a variety of environments within his or her daily routine. Often, the functional assessment may take a few visits to complete.

For an older adult with a visual impairment, activities of daily living are key to the person's living situation. If the older adult is not able to perform critical activities of daily living, he or she may need a more supportive living environment. For that reason, the O&M specialist will incorporate routes and orientation skills that are related to these daily living skills.

Home environment: The O&M specialist is able to assess the older adult in his or her home. Included in this assessment is a careful observation of potential fall risks such as unsecured area rugs, uneven surfaces, objects on the floor, etc. The O&M specialist should also note if the older adult is able to negotiate all areas of the home, for example, the bathroom, bedroom, social areas, yard, and if he or she is able to retrieve the mail.

Residential environment: The residential assessment may include routes to various areas in the person's neighborhood. This can include travel to a friend's house, church, or nearby store. If the older adult lives in a senior community, the residential environment is combined with the home environment.

Semi-business environment: The semi-business environment is usually more complicated and may involve public transportation. The older adult with visual impairment may be interested in accessing community leisure areas and traveling to destinations outside their home or residential area.

Business environment: Many older adults may desire to travel into (or live in) urban environments that are typically complicated and visually complex. There may be crowded situations as well as noisier surroundings.

All environments: The O&M specialist should consider personal safety concerns in each of these environments. Personal safety refers to having a backup plan, alternate route, or another assistance option in place in case of an emergency. This may include pre-programmed numbers on a cell phone or noting stores that are open during the time the person is traveling that might be a safe haven. The alternate routes are also individualized to the abilities of each older adult. A person who moves at a slow pace will need more time to avoid or escape a dangerous situation (Bozeman, 2004).

Environmental considerations: Since environments are dynamic, finding the optimal conditions with regard to lighting, contrast, and size (of objects or text) can be daunting. There is also an overlap between these conditions. For example, changes in lighting may increase the need for better contrast or a change in size needed for the client to identify objects and visual clues. Lighting, contrast, and size requirements will vary according to the task. For example, an older adult may require increased contrast if the lighting is poor in an area or require larger lettering on street signs if the contrast is not good.

Lighting, contrast, and size can all be increased or decreased depending on the task that needs to be carried out. When adjusting lighting, problem lighting and glare should be considered, as well as transitions from dim to bright conditions and vice versa. For contrast, some colors, such as red on green, may be problematic, while other options, such as yellow on black, may work better. Visual clutter or a busy background may be difficult for the older adult with visual impairment as well. With size, bigger is not always better. If the older adult has a significant field restriction, a smaller object within the field of view may be better to use than a larger one since more of the object can be viewed.

SUMMARY

Sensory changes are a normal part of the aging process. It is important to keep in mind the effect these changes can have on O&M instruction for older clients with visual impairments. Careful assessment and a client-directed approach that integrates the goals and passions of the older adult will support long-term progress.

With any rehabilitation process there are many professionals with expertise in different areas who work with the older adult with visual impairment. Often, occupational therapists, physical therapists, and orientation and mobility specialists, along with other professionals, comprise the team that supports the older adult with vision loss. Integrating the expertise of these team members is important to the functional outcomes for the older client. Collaboration and teamwork cannot be underestimated. More information about collaboration is provided in Chapter 8.

LEARNING ACTIVITIES

1. Look at the medications your parent or grandparent takes. Research the effects each medication has on all five senses. Make a list of the side effects.

2. Consider the more common sensory and physical changes that occur with aging. These may include stiff joints due to arthritis, diminished hearing and vision abilities, and reduced tactile abilities. Develop an activity for a small group of co-workers or fellow students in which one or more of these changes are simulated. Be creative! A ruler may be taped on the elbow or knee to limit movement of the joint; ear plugs can reduce hearing; making a mask with several layers of plastic wrap and securing it with masking tape around the wearer's head can blur vision; wearing gloves can reduce tactile abilities. Have them participate in specific tasks to test the simulated changes; for example, bending down to retrieve dropped objects, listening to a phone call, reading the directions on a medicine bottle, or dialing a phone number. Discuss the challenges and overall perceptions.

3. Choose a health disorder common in older adults (such as diabetes, osteoarthritis, or neuropathy). Make a list of how the disorder can affect the daily routine of an older adult with visual impairment. Reflect on instructional strategies that might address the items on the list. For example, think about setting the table, going to the store, getting the mail, and visiting friends.

References

Boyce, J. M., & Shone, G. R. (2006). The effects of ageing on smell and taste. *Postgraduate Medical Journal, 82*(966), 239–241.

Bozeman, L. A. (2004). Environmental and personal safety: No vision required [Practice Report]. *Journal of Visual Impairment & Blindness, 98*(7), 434–438.

Bozeman, L. A., & Bozeman, J. K. (n.d.). Unpublished manuscript.

Chittka, L., & Brockmann, A. (2005). Perception space—The final frontier. *PLoS Biology, 3*(4), e137.

Colenbrander, A. (2009). The functional classification of brain damage-related vision loss. *Journal of Visual Impairment & Blindness, 103*(2), 118–123.

Crews, J. E., & Campbell, V. A. (2004). Vision impairment and hearing loss among community-dwelling older Americans: Implications for health and functioning. *American Journal of Public Health, 94*(5), 823–829.

Dillon, H. (2001). *Hearing aids.* Sydney, Australia: Boomerang Press.

DiSogra, R. M., & Weir, K. (1993). The side effects of drugs on hearing, auditory perception and other related systems. *Audiololgy Today, 5*(6), 30–35.

Fagerström, R. (1994). Self-image of elderly persons before and after cataract surgery. *Journal of Visual Impairment & Blindness, 88*(5), 458–461.

Faye, E. E. (1984). *Clinical low vision* (2nd ed.). Boston: Little Brown and Co.

Fuller, G. F. (2000). Falls in the elderly. *American Family Physician, 61*(7), 2159–2168, 2173–2174.

Geruschat, D. R., & De l'Aune, W. (1989). Reliability and validity of O&M instructor observations. *Journal of Visual Impairment & Blindness, 83*(9), 457–460.

Griffin-Shirley, N., & Welsh, R. L. (2010). Teaching orientation and mobility to older adults. In W. R. Wiener, R. L. Welsh, & B. B. Blasch (Eds.), *Foundations of orientation and mobility: Vol. II. Instructional strategies and practical applications* (3rd ed., pp. 286–308). New York: AFB Press.

Johnson, J. A., Cox, R. M., & Alexander, G. C. (2010). Development of APHAB norms for WDRC hearing aids and comparisons with original norms. *Ear and Hearing, 31*(1), 47–55.

Kerkhoff, G. (2000). Neurovisual rehabilitation: Recent developments and future directions. *Journal of Neurology, Neurosurgery & Psychiatry, 68,* 691–706.

Koutsoklenis, A., & Papadopoulos, K. (2011). Olfactory cues used for wayfinding in urban environments by individuals with visual impairments. *Journal of Visual Impairment & Blindness, 105*(10), 692–702.

Lawson, G. D., & Wiener, W. R. (2010). Audition for students with vision loss. In W. R. Wiener, R. L. Welsh, & B. B. Blasch (Eds.), *Foundations of orientation and mobility: Vol. I. History and theory* (3rd ed., pp. 84–136). New York: AFB Press.

Milligan, K. (1998). Mobility options for visually impaired persons with diabetes: Considerations for orientation and mobility instructors. *Journal of Visual Impairment & Blindness, 92*(1), 71–79.

Mogk, L. G., & Mogk, M. (2003). *Macular degeneration: The complete guide to saving and maximizing your sight.* New York: Ballantine Publishing Group.

Orr, A. L., & Rogers, P. (2006). *Aging and vision loss: A handbook for families.* New York: AFB Press.

Ponchillia, S. V. (1993). Complications of diabetes and their implications for service providers. *Journal of Visual Impairment & Blindness, 87*(9), 354–358.

Riddering, A. T. (2008). Keeping older adults with vision loss safe: Chronic conditions and comorbidities that influence functional mobility. *Journal of Visual Impairment & Blindness, 102*(10), 616–620.

Rosen, S., & Crawford, J. S. (2010). Teaching orientation and mobility to learners with visual, physical, and health impairments. In W. R. Wiener, R. L. Welsh, &

B. B. Blasch (Eds.), *Foundations of orientation and mobility: Vol. II. Instructional strategies and practical applications* (3rd ed., pp. 564–623). New York: AFB Press.

Sense. (2013). *Deafblindness and other senses.* Retrieved from http://www.sense.org.uk/content/deafblindness-and-other-senses

Shinn, J. B. (2012). An overview of (central) auditory processing disorders. *Audiology Online.* Retrieved from http://www.audiologyonline.com/articles/overview-central-auditory-processing-disorders-782

Vaupel, J. W. (2010). Biodemography of human ageing [Electronic version]. *Nature, 464,* 536–542. Retrieved from http://www.nature.com/nature/journal/v464/n7288/full/nature08984.html

Vukicevic, M., & Fitzmaurice, K. (2008). Butterflies and black lacy patterns: The prevalence and characteristics of Charles Bonnet hallucinations in an Australian population. *Clinical & Experimental Ophthalmology, 36*(7), 659–665.

Warren, M. (2008). Memory loss, dementia, and stroke: Implications for rehabilitation of older adults with age-related macular degeneration. *Journal of Visual Impairment & Blindness, 102*(10), 611–615.

Working Group on Auditory Processing Disorders. (2005). *(Central) auditory processing disorders* [Technical report]. Rockville, MD: American Speech-Language-Hearing Association. Retrieved from http://www.asha.org/policy/tr2005-00043.htm

CHAPTER 3

Modifying Orientation and Mobility Techniques for Older Adults with Visual Impairments

Anita Page and Laura Bozeman

This chapter covers modifications to basic orientation and mobility (O&M) skills that are useful when teaching older adults with visual impairments. These skills—such as guiding and protective techniques, trailing, room familiarization, and search patterns—play an important role in helping older clients retain independence and increase safety. The standard versions of these skills have been well documented and are widely used throughout the O&M profession, and have proved to be very useful to people with visual impairment in moving within their environments with increased safety and efficiency.

As the O&M profession develops and grows to include training for a more diverse population, modifications are created for clients who are not able to use the standard methods. (For a complete description of the standard method of teaching these basic O&M skills, see Hill & Ponder, 1976; Jacobson, 2013; LaGrow & Long, 2011.) Not only do O&M professionals need to be open to making modifications to techniques in order to accommodate the older population, they need to be flexible in their approach and initial contact with older adults. Older adults come from different cultures, have varied backgrounds, and have developed skills from different experiences throughout their life. It is important for an O&M specialist to value these characteristics and consider the benefits these qualities bring to the training plan and subsequent instruction. Integrating these aspects when first meeting with an older adult is critical to establishing a quality rapport. Successful preparation is illustrated in the Appendix at the end of this chapter, which describes the experiences of an O&M specialist teaching older rural Alaskans with visual impairments.

WORKING WITH AN OLDER CLIENT

Modifications to O&M techniques may be used to address balance problems, physical weakness, hearing, or cognitive issues. Older adults who have visual impairments often have additional physical, cognitive, or emotional challenges that require modifications in how a basic O&M skill is taught and how the older adult will use the skill. It is the responsibility of the O&M specialist to assess the older adult to determine when a modification would be helpful and how to modify the skill. The specialist must carefully weigh any change in the performance of the skill that might result from a modification, and ensure that the safety of the client is not compromised as a result of a modification. Successful modification allows older adults to get the maximum benefit when utilizing O&M skills, and helps them maintain some level of independence, even if they are not able to perform a standard O&M technique.

It is important to build rapport and gain the trust of older adults "because orientation and mobility is taught using a one-on-one teaching approach and the process frequently involves the confronting of various psychosocial barriers and significant personal challenges by the student, the relationship that develops between the student and the instructor is especially important." (Welsh, 2010, p. 140). Many older clients may still be dealing with the emotional shock of vision loss as well as other issues of aging and may need time to prepare for and process instruction in O&M skills. Find out how much the older adult knows about his or her eye disease and spend time educating him or her if necessary. Listen carefully to older individuals to discover their concerns about their vision loss as well as what interests they have and if they have discontinued any activities due to the loss of vision. This is valuable information that can be used when developing an individualized orientation and mobility program.

When interacting with older adults, it is important for the O&M specialist to consider clients' perspective about their visual condition. They may hold negative perceptions of vision loss (known as the stigma of blindness) that are still common in society—for example, that a person who is blind is not capable of autonomous action or that blindness itself is a shameful condition. Many factors, such as geographical location, the era in which the individual grew up, personal experiences, and cultural beliefs, may influence the development of such a stigmatized view of blindness. For some individuals, their ideas of what blindness is can be deeply ingrained and difficult to overcome.

Misconceptions held by the older adult, or by society in general, can be more debilitating than the blindness itself. An individual who believes that blindness is something to be ashamed of and that people with vision loss cannot be self-sufficient has erected a serious barrier to learning the skills necessary to become independent. "The most formidable barrier with which blind people must cope is not the physical loss of sight. It is, rather, the myths, misconceptions, negative attitudes, and stereotypes about blindness" (Benson, n.d., p. 8). Because they do not want to appear helpless or vulnerable, some older adults will try to conceal their visual impairment from the public. Resistance or reluctance to begin a training program can often stem from the simple fact that a client will no longer be able to conceal his or her visual impairment once he or she begins to use a cane. It is important to address negative attitudes about blindness so that the client is more willing to engage in training. All of these concerns should be acknowledged so the older adult knows the instructor has "heard" his or her feelings. Offering examples of accomplishments or scenarios about the successes of people with visual impairments may allow the older adult to relate and gain a new perspective. As O&M instruction continues, most older adults begin to develop a sense of accomplishment and confidence, which can encourage them to want to do more. Listening to the older client is critically important to building rapport.

The older adult's feelings and views should always be taken into account (Griffin-Shirley & Welsh, 2010). Feeling "heard" can build trust and foster a two-way approach—the client and the instructor working together—to the older adult's O&M instruction. The older adult should always be involved in the development of his or her own O&M program. Family, friends, and support personnel also play a crucial role in providing support and helping older adults maintain the level of independence that they desire, and it is important for them to be included whenever possible in the planning and implementation of any O&M program. This involvement fosters more effective reinforcement of skills and expectations within the older adult's daily routine.

COMMUNICATION BETWEEN GUIDE AND TRAVELER

Some people feel more secure when they receive verbal reinforcement of the sensory information they perceive when being guided by another person, whether an O&M specialist or a friend or family member. When a guide verbally acknowledges, for example, a change in walking surface from tile to carpet, or identifies a sound as it occurs ("Josie is passing us with her walker"), this can make the traveler feel more confident in his or her interpretation of the environment. To help the older adult learn to differentiate sounds, the O&M specialist may also point out, for example, when the nurse is passing with the medication cart and talk about how the cart sounds different than Josie and her walker.

Communication skills are essential for safe and effective guidance. It is important that clients with visual impairments express their needs to their guides. When working with an inexperienced guide, the older adult may need to demonstrate a basic technique with any corresponding modifications so the guide can understand how he or she is used to traveling. The traveler should feel comfortable stating a preferred side or asking for a greater or lesser degree of verbal description of the environment as he/she travels. It is the O&M specialist's responsibility to help a client learn the best way to communicate his or her needs and reach the desired level of independence and comfort.

The rest of this chapter covers specific O&M techniques and ways in which they may be modified for older adults, including basic guiding techniques, personal protective techniques, trailing, seating, search patterns, room familiarization, and negotiating cars. A brief introduction to the long white cane is also included, as well as safety considerations for working with older clients. (Please note that to avoid the use of awkward language when describing specific techniques, for the purposes of this chapter we will assume the O&M specialist is a woman and the older adult client is a man.)

GUIDING TECHNIQUES

Guiding techniques refer essentially to human guide techniques, or methods in which a person who is visually impaired uses the assistance of another individual for orientation. The standard method of guiding a person with a visual impairment is to have the traveler grasp the guide's arm just above the elbow, keeping the traveler's arm bent at approximately a 90-degree angle (Griffin-Shirley & Groff, 1993). The bend in the traveler's arm helps maintain a half-step distance behind the guide and provides a brace for stops.

Jacobson (2013) states, "The human guide procedures lay the foundation for building a trusting relationship and a positive rapport between the O&M specialist and student" (p. 86). If the traveler is attentive, he or she can learn

Modifying Orientation and Mobility Techniques 49

a lot about the guide as soon as he or she contacts the guide's elbow. Did the traveler have to reach up or down to grasp the elbow? This is a good indicator of the height of the guide. Is the elbow soft, supple, muscular, or bony? Any of these traits may indicate the age and sex of the guide. A sense of fear and indecision from a new guide or calm confidence from an experienced guide may even be transferred through the elbow to the hand of the traveler (Gallagher, 1974). Presenting instruction in guiding techniques in a confident, relaxed manner will facilitate the process of building rapport.

The interaction during the initial instruction in guiding techniques is the best time for the O&M specialist to establish a rapport and trust with the client by developing good communication and demonstrating dedication to the client's success. Instruction ought to occur in a quiet area with good lighting and no background noise or distractions. The O&M specialist will want to determine if the client can hear the instruction and whether the client's hearing is better on one side than the other. The O&M specialist should position herself on the same level as the client and face him when speaking. The O&M specialist should speak clearly and not talk down to the client by oversimplifying the instructions as if the task is too difficult for the older adult to understand. If the older adult has a hearing impairment, it may take a little longer for him to process and respond to what is being said. This delay should not be mistaken for a cognitive issue. After completing the instructions, the specialist should check the client's understanding by having him restate the objective of the lesson. This will give the specialist an indication of how much information the client can retain at a time. If the client is confused or cannot remember what was said, the specialist may need to break each skill down into its individual steps.

To provide extra support for a client with balance issues, the guide can bend her arm at a 90-degree angle and the traveler can grasp the guide's forearm instead of the point above the elbow (see Figure 3.1). This grip provides additional support. Using this grip will decrease the distance between the guide and traveler, which limits the reaction time of the traveler. However, the walking pace is usually slower, which allows the pair more time to react.

The guide may also interlock the fingers of her guiding arm with those of the traveler to further modify this grip (see Figure 3.2).

For even more support, the traveler can grasp the guide's arm with both hands (Jacobson, 2013, p. 107). This modification provides the benefit of extra support, but at the cost of reaction time, since this position places the

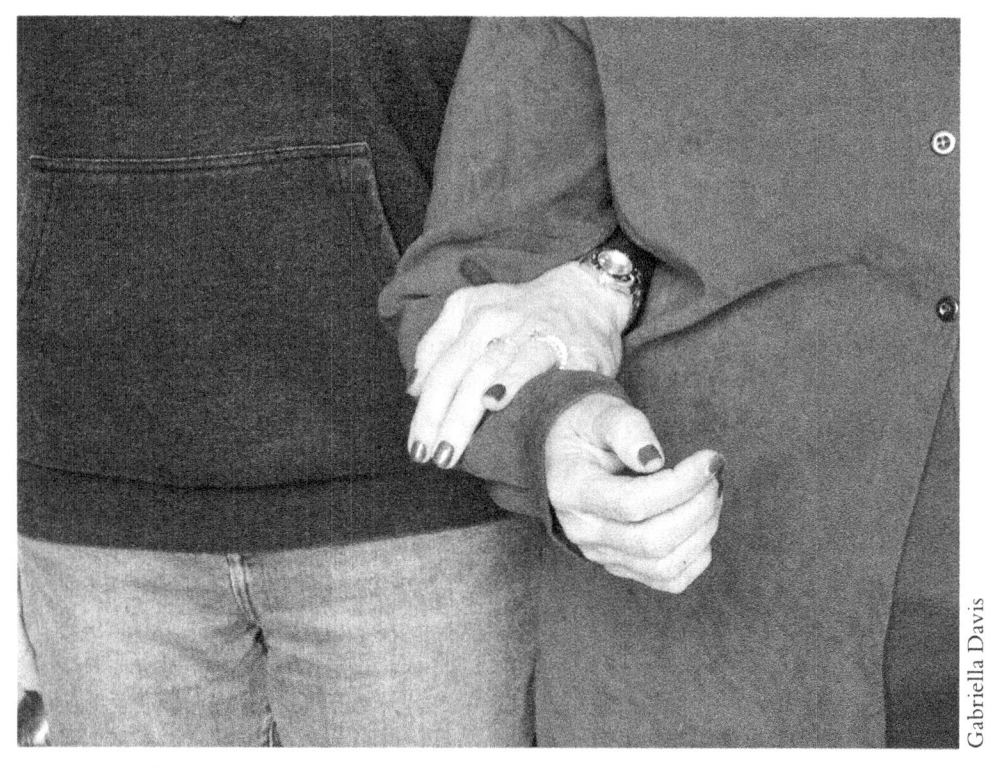

FIGURE **3.1**
Grip for human guide modified to provide extra support for clients with balance issues. The guide (right) bends her arm at a 90-degree angle. The traveler (left) grasps the guide's forearm.

individual at the side of the guide rather than a half-step behind. When using this position, the guide will also need to move at a slower pace and modify her movements in order to clear the width of two people around obstacles to ensure safe travel.

It is always best to walk at the pace of the slower member of the team. Sometimes people travel very slowly and pull back out of fear or lack of trust in their guides. It can be scary the first few times that a person ventures out of his or her comfort zone. If they also have very little experience being guided, they may become anxious. Even when a person is comfortable using guiding techniques, he or she may be cautious with a new person guiding him/her. If fear or a lack of trust is the reason for the slower pace, then once the traveler is familiar with guiding techniques and the person guiding them, their pace should increase. This is another reason O&M specialists will want to priori-

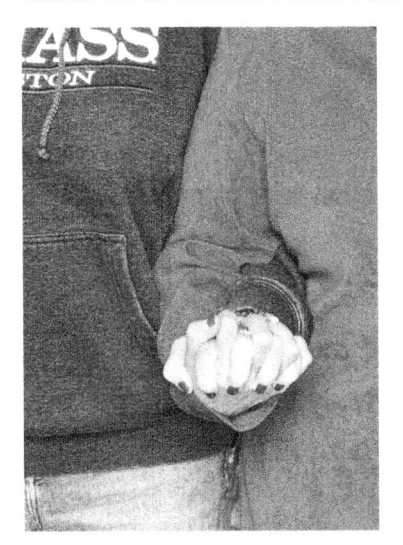

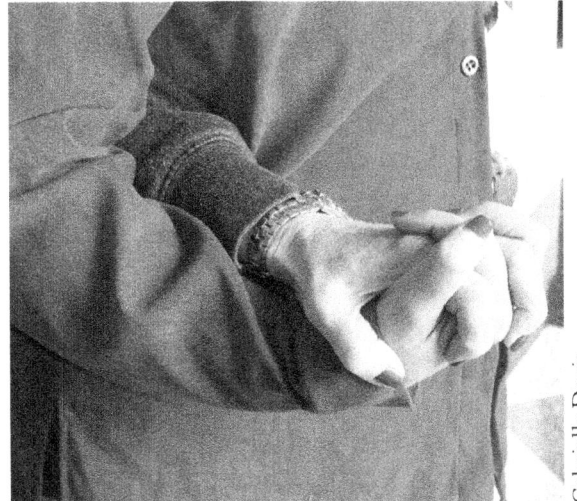

Modifying Orientation and Mobility Techniques 51

FIGURE **3.2**
Front view (left) and side view (right) of a support grip with interlocking fingers.

tize establishing rapport and developing trust with their clients. It should be noted that balance problems can occur when traveling at a very slow pace, but the problem usually corrects itself once the client is comfortable with the guide and the team can travel at the client's normal pace. If a change in pace is detected, it is important for the O&M specialist to question the older adult to find out what is causing the change. A slower pace may be due to pain, dizziness, confusion, or fear, among other reasons. These issues should be addressed before continuing with the training.

Reversing Directions

To turn around and continue traveling in the opposite direction, one member of the team will usually initiate the action by stating the need to go back. The standard method has the team complete the following sequence:

1. Stop.
2. Traveler and guide turn 90 degrees to face each other.
3. Traveler finds the guide's free elbow with his free hand and grasps it.
4. Traveler releases his original grasp.
5. Traveler and guide turn another 90 degrees, to face the opposite direction.

The guide can facilitate step 3 by contacting the traveler's free hand with the back of her free hand so that the free elbow can be easily found.

If the traveler has balance issues, this procedure should be done slowly. The guide may stop and have the traveler lean against a wall or hold on to a chair while the guide helps reestablish the traveler's grip on the other side. This modification allows the traveler to have some support at the point the grip needs to change.

Transferring Sides

Sometimes there is a need for the traveler to move to the other side of the guide, such as when approaching doors or stairways (as described later in this section). The action can be initiated by either team member. Usually the traveler makes this change by walking behind the guide, maintaining physical contact, and reestablishing the grip on the other side. This switch can be done in a static position or while traveling. If the traveler has balance issues, it is best if the guide comes to a stop before the switch happens. As a modification, the guide can move to the other side while maintaining physical contact with the traveler.

Narrow Passageways

When approaching a crowded area or a narrow passageway, the guide moves the guiding arm to the small of her back, which indicates to the traveler that they are approaching an area that requires a single-file formation for safe passage. To facilitate this change, the traveler extends the arm that is grasping the guide, slides his hand to the guide's wrist, and moves directly behind the guide, so that they take up the width of only one person. The extension of the traveler's arm keeps him from walking on the guide's heels. A traveler with balance difficulties may need to hold on to the guide's wrist with both hands.

Negotiating Doors

The narrow passage position facilitates going through a doorway safely. The guide tells the traveler the direction of the door's swing (toward or away from the pair) and to which side the door opens, so that the traveler can have the hand on that side free to catch the door. This may require the traveler to switch sides as the pair approaches the door. The guide opens the door and moves first through the doorway. The traveler is expected to catch the door and close it behind him if necessary. This can also be done without switching sides by approaching the door in narrow passageway position. From this position it is easy for the traveler to free up the hand needed to catch the door by switching which hand holds the guide's arm, if necessary, and then resuming the original position once they have passed through the door.

Self-closing doors can present a problem for older adults who may not have the strength to hold the weight of the door. Because the older traveler may be slow moving, the guide cannot simply give the door a good push so that they both clear the opening before it closes. To modify this technique, the following sequence can be used:

1. The guide opens the door.
2. The guide rests the open door on her hip.
3. The guide turns to face the traveler, so that the guide's back is toward the direction of travel.
4. The guide bends her arms at the elbows with the forearms rotated so that the hands are palm up. The traveler grasps both of the guide's arms with his hands on top of the guide's forearms.
5. The guide maintains contact with the door and rotates 90 degrees away from the door as the traveler steps through and clears the opening of the door.
6. The guide has the traveler release the arm farthest from the door as the guide rotates another 90 degrees to face the original direction of travel, with the door now resting on the guide's opposite hip.
7. The guide then steps forward, clearing the door and allowing it to close, and the pair resumes their travels.

Stairs

Using the standard method of navigating stairs, the guide announces to the traveler that they are approaching an ascending or descending staircase, faces the stairs, and approaches them squarely, bringing the traveler up to the first step so that the traveler's toes are either touching the riser for ascending stairs or right on the edge for descending stairs. If there is a handrail, the traveler should be positioned so he can use it, which may require switching sides. The guide will take the first step and the traveler will follow, staying one step behind the guide. When the guide reaches the landing, the guide will pause to indicate that the traveler will also reach the landing after the next step.

Although the normal gait when traversing stairs is to ascend or descend the staircase with each step, an older adult who has arthritis, weakness, extra weight, or balance issues may need to place both feet on each step before taking the next step. If the client is at risk of falling, a gait belt can be used to provide additional safety (Rosen & Crawford, 2010). A gait belt is a device that has the appearance of an oversized wide belt, usually made of a cotton-webbed material, and a buckle. Gait belts may be obtained at any store that sells medical supplies or online (Rosen & Crawford, 2010). A gait belt is used as a safety measure when transferring people with mobility, weakness, or balance issues from one position to another and while helping people who are recovering from surgery or who have weakness or balance issues improve their gait (gait training). When used correctly, the gait belt can protect the person wearing it from falls and the person holding it from hurting his or her back. If used incorrectly, a gait belt can cause injury. O&M specialists need to work with a physical therapist or nurse to learn the correct way to use a gait belt.

SELF-PROTECTIVE TECHNIQUES

Protective techniques are designed to provide protection for the individual with a visual impairment while he or she is moving independently through the environment. Generally, these techniques are used to detect obstacles at waist height, such as furniture and countertops, or at head and shoulder height, such as cabinets, open doors, or low-hanging tree branches. These techniques can be used while traveling independently in open spaces to locate anticipated landmarks and to detect and avoid potential problems. The upper protective technique should also be used when bending over to protect the face and head. The techniques can also be used in conjunction with other techniques or tools to facilitate safe travel.

Upper Protective Technique

The upper protective technique is used, as the name implies, to provide protection for the head and chest. It requires the ability to raise the arm to shoulder level, parallel to the floor, and bend the elbow to bring the forearm across the upper portion of the body. In the correct position, the shoulder is flexed and the upper arm extended forward with a 90-degree angle between the upper arm and torso, and the elbow is extended at about 120 degrees, bringing the hand about a foot in front of the opposite shoulder with the palm facing out

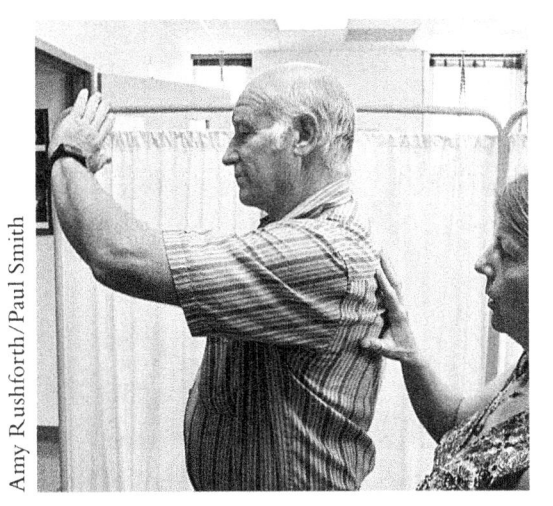

FIGURE **3.3**

Man using upper protective technique with correct posture.

(Rushforth, 2009; see Figure 3.3). The hand provides protection for the opposite shoulder or the forearm can be raised to protect the face. If not done correctly, this technique can cause tension and fatigue, and may result in overuse injuries and secondary orthopedic issues. If the older client is taught to use the correct position for the upper protective technique, such issues can be avoided.

When assuming the upper protective technique, elevating the scapula (shoulder blade) before lifting the arm, as shown in Figure 3.4A (Rushforth, 2009), will result in injury to the shoulder. Therefore, the O&M specialist will want to keep an eye out for this type of posture and provide correction immediately. To help the client position his shoulder correctly, the O&M specialist can first place one hand on the client's scapula and one on the front of the shoulder, as shown in Figure 3.4B. The next step is to lift the shoulder upward, as shown in Figure 3.4C, to make the client aware of what it feels like when the shoulder is held too high. This example should help the older adult be able to detect when his shoulder is tense and allow him to correct the position. Then, the O&M specialist asks the client to drop his shoulder all the way down (see Figure 3.4D). In this position, the client's scapula is stable. Keeping the scapula in the stable position, the client can then lift his arm and position it properly for self-protection (Rushforth, 2009). This position (shown in Figure 3.3) should help prevent fatigue and other potential injuries.

If clients have arthritis or other orthopedic conditions that prohibit them from performing a part or all of the movements necessary for the proper upper protective technique, modifications can be made to enable protection while traveling. Wearing a hat with a wide brim can help indicate when a

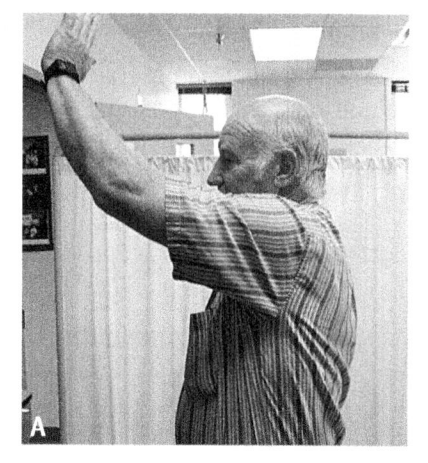

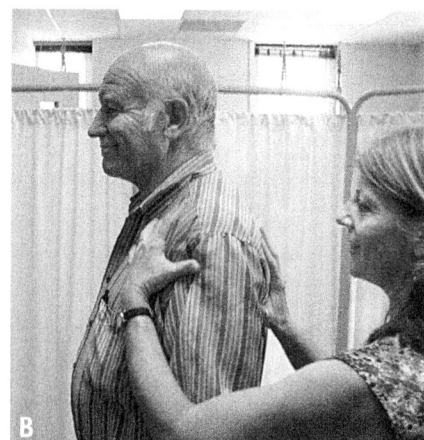

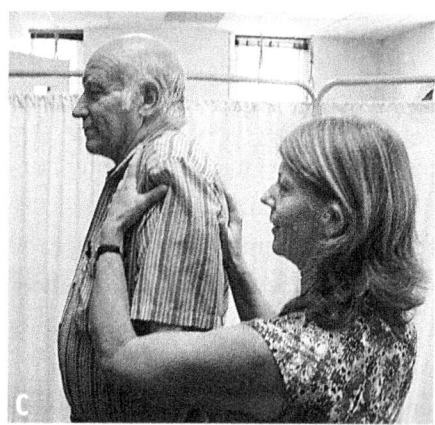

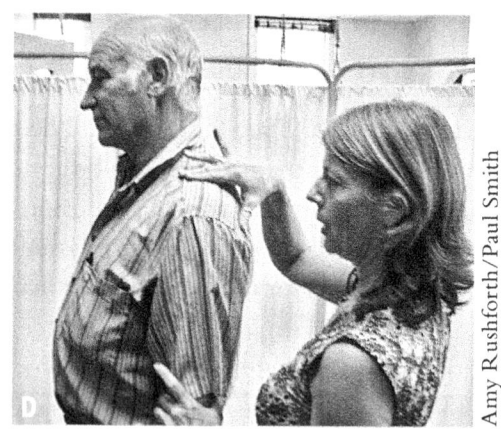

FIGURE **3.4**

(A) A man using upper protective technique with incorrect posture; his shoulder is raised. **(B)** The O&M specialist provides guidance on proper positioning by placing one hand on the man's shoulder blade and the other hand in front of his shoulder. **(C)** The O&M specialist keeps her hands on the man's shoulder blade and in front of his shoulder as he lifts his shoulder. **(D)** The man stands with shoulder lowered and a stable, correctly positioned shoulder blade.

client's head is about to come into contact with an object. Another simple modification is to have older adults carry an object in their hand that is anywhere from 6 to 24 inches in length and light enough for them to hold to extend their reach and area of protection. Examples of appropriate objects are a folded-up long cane, a reacher (a long stick-like tool, sometimes also called a grabber, which extends an individual's reach and enables him or her to pick up objects with the jaw-like end), a rolled-up magazine, a newspaper, or an umbrella. This modification extends the client's sensory reach while allowing his arm to remain in a lower, easier-to-maintain position.

Lower Protective Technique

The lower protective technique provides protection from waist-high obstacles such as dressers, couches, or tables. To perform this technique, the client places a hand approximately 12 inches in front of the opposite hip, with the palm facing the body. The space between the hand and the body acts as a bumper. When obstacles are contacted by the extended hand or arm, the client has a little extra time to stop moving forward before contacting the obstacle with the rest of the body. As with the upper protective technique, if a client has difficulty reaching across the body, a newspaper, long shoe horn, back scratcher, or other lightweight object can extend the reach.

Using protective techniques while traveling independently does not provide the types of information that traveling with a guide (human or dog) or a long white cane does, such as changes in terrain or potential ground-level stumbling hazards. The use of a shopping cart or other ambulatory device, such as a walker, can also provide a limited preview of the terrain, or detection of low-lying obstacles in time to enable an appropriate response to maintain safe travel. See Chapter 4 for more information about canes and other mobility tools.

TRAILING A WALL

Trailing is a technique that involves maintaining constant contact with a parallel surface, frequently a wall that shows the direction of travel. Trailing helps the individual who is visually impaired maintain proper direction and locate things found along the wall, such as a door, hallway, or elevator. The standard techniques for trailing along a wall (as described in the texts of Hill & Ponder, 1976; Jacobson, 2013; and LaGrow & Long, 2011) require that some part of the hand or fingers lightly touch the wall's surface. If an older client has very delicate skin, neuropathy, or painful joints, the O&M specialist can modify this technique by having the older adult wear a glove to protect the trailing hand or contact the wall with something lightweight, such as a rolled-up newspaper or a pen. If it is too difficult for the client to maintain constant contact with the wall, the client can instead contact the wall every few steps to verify his or her position. (Trailing can also be done with a cane, a more advanced technique, if the client uses one.)

SEATING

It is important to give accurate information about the seating arrangement when guiding an older adult to a chair. Be sure to include whether or not the chair has arms, the height of the chair, if it swivels or has wheels. Is it near a table, and if so, where is the table? Make sure to include information about people in the area and where are they located.

Using the standard guiding position, approach the chair so that the older adult is facing the seat of the chair and have them step forward so that they can feel the chair with the front of their legs. The client should then use the upper protective technique (modified with the elbow in, touching the torso, positioning the hand in front of the face) while reaching down with the other hand, palm side up, to clear the seat, turn, and sit down. This process can be done in one smooth motion. Modified upper protective technique is used any time the person bends forward. The seat is cleared to prevent sitting on an object. If the chair cannot be approached head on, then the guide needs to bring the client to the chair and place his hand on the chair. The traveler can then follow the guide's arm down to the chair. The guide should describe to the older adult the position of the chair and where they are in relation to it, such as, "this is the back of the chair."

It is important to take into consideration the seating preference of an older client. Clients know what works best for them in terms of type of seating arrangement, type of chair, and type of lighting they need for best visual functioning. The O&M specialist can teach individuals who have some usable vision to systematically scan the environment for available seating and to direct their guide to where they want to go. For individuals who are blind, a guide may describe the type of seating available and where it is located; for example, is it in a crowded, noisy area or quiet and secluded? If the individual has a hearing impairment, the guide may need to be careful to avoid seating near a main entrance, overhead vents, speakers, or areas with noticeable echo.

Older adults who have difficulty getting in and out of chairs will most likely have a preference for straight-backed chairs with arms that can provide some leverage when rising from the seated position. Such clients can be encouraged to move their hips to the front of the chair and use their leg muscles to stand up (National Osteoporosis Foundation, n.d.). If the client has a lot of difficulty getting in and out of chairs, refer him or her to a physical therapist for an evaluation (Rosen & Crawford, 2010).

SEARCH PATTERNS

Learning how to look for something that has been dropped is a basic O&M technique. The standard technique when a client drops an object is to first listen to try to determine in which direction the object fell or rolled, then walk in that direction. At the point where the individual thinks the object may have settled, he or she squats down, keeping the back straight, or gets on hands and knees to begin searching. Systematic search patterns, such as linear, fan, or the expanding box, are taught to make sure the area is searched comprehensively (Hill & Ponder, 1976; Jacobson, 2013; LaGrow & Long, 2011).

Older clients with balance issues may need to hold on to something stable (if available) when moving to the floor to search for the dropped object. If squatting down or getting onto hands and knees is too difficult, a client may remain standing and use his feet to search for the object or use a broom and dustpan in a systematic fashion to sweep up the dropped object. If a footstool is available, the client may find it easier to sit on the stool and conduct the search using his feet. A vacuum cleaner can also be a useful tool for locating small objects such as a pill or hearing aid battery if the opening is covered so the object is not sucked down the hose. The client can use a rubber band to secure the leg of a pair of pantyhose over the opening of a vacuum hose and vacuum the area where the object was dropped. The object will be held to the surface of the pantyhose until the vacuum is turned off (Carleyy, n.d.). As always, the upper protective technique should be employed to protect the head any time the individual bends forward.

If a client frequently drops the same type of object, such as his medication or hearing aid battery, a change in his routine might be necessary. For example, if he consistently drops his medication, the O&M specialist might suggest that he always be seated when he takes his medication. If the client has some remaining vision, the medication can be placed on a tray that contrasts well against the surface where he will be seated so that the client can see where he needs to reach. The tray can also be lined with felt or another fabric that will keep the objects in place. The same techniques can be used for preparing to change a hearing aid battery. Keeping the hands free when walking can greatly reduce the number of objects a client will drop. Adding pockets, aprons, or baskets to walkers will keep items within reach and convenient, and will leave the hands free.

ROOM FAMILIARIZATION

Once the trailing technique has been mastered and can be carried out safely, older adults with visual impairments can learn the techniques used to familiarize themselves with an unknown room or area. In the room familiarization technique, the client usually starts with the wall to the right of the door. He trails the wall and then assigns a label to it—such as "medication wall" because his medications are kept in a cabinet on that wall—to help him remember the wall when he returns to the starting point. Once each wall is trailed and named and the client is comfortable with the perimeter, the interior of the room is explored, usually using a systematic grid pattern.

If the client has low vision, the room can be scanned visually before starting the familiarization process. As the perimeter is trailed, the client can use his vision to gather more information. Using high contrast at key points such as light switches and doorways can increase their visibility, making them easier to find. When teaching this technique, it can be helpful to have the client narrate aloud what he sees. This allows the O&M specialist to have a glimpse of what the client can see and if he is able to correctly identify and interpret visual information.

Clients who use wheelchairs or walkers can still use the room familiarization technique. An adult who uses a wheelchair can trail the wall as he is being pushed or, if he pushes himself, can stop and explore the wall between pushes. The method can also be used with walkers. (Wheelchairs and walkers are discussed in detail in Chapter 4.)

Identification of landmarks that are meaningful to the individual and tactile maps can be helpful when someone is learning a new environment. For example, in a gym, one person may want to know where the stationary bikes are in the workout area while another person is only interested in the sauna. These two individuals will chose different landmarks within the gym based on their importance to the route (making the landmark easier to remember) and that will help them reach their destination. When creating a tactile map, have the student chose the tactile marker that he or she would like to use for the different landmarks on the map. One person may chose a round button for the stationary bike while another person may chose a marker that is soft and squishy, like the feel of the bicycle seat. (More information about making tactile maps and teaching with maps can be found in Bentzen & Marston, 2010; Pogrund et al., 2012.)

Remembering the layout of a new room or area can be a challenge for some clients. Every person has a learning style that suits him or her best. For clients with memory issues, a recording device can be used to record the description. Additional strategies that may be helpful for memory and retention are rehearsal, association, categorization, mnemonics, and visualization (Griffin-Shirley & Welsh, 2010, p. 299). The *rehearsal* strategy uses repetition to help with memory. Using this strategy requires people with visual impairment to go through the room familiarization process several times. The process may need to be broken down and each wall of the room reviewed several times before moving on to the next wall. Speaking aloud (parallel talk) about what is contacted as the wall is trailed and repeating it is also rehearsal (Bozeman & McCulley, 2010).

To use the *association* strategy with the room familiarization process, the O&M specialist begins in a comfortable and familiar area and slowly expands the area to include new environments. The *categorization* strategy can help the older adult make a connection between a place and its function by first labeling a room (such as the bedroom) and then having the older adult think of all the things usually found in that type of room (a bed, a dresser, a chair, a closet) before embarking on room familiarization. This strategy prepares the client for what to expect when exploring the room and can shift the focus to the layout of the room rather than identification of objects and surfaces.

The use of *mnemonics* can be a fun way to remember landmarks inside a room. For example, as a client named Sally walks the perimeter of her kitchen, she contacts the counter, followed by the sink, a door, the oven, and finally the refrigerator. She assigns each one of those things a letter (*C* for counter, *S* for sink, *D* for door, *O* for oven, and *F* for fridge) and comes up with a kitchen-related saying that uses the first letter of each landmark in order, such as "Chef Sally delivers our food."

Once the room familiarization process is complete, *visualization* can be used to reinforce the new information. Have the older adult sit in the room, point to each wall, and describe what she discovered as she explored each wall. If possible, this procedure should be done from different positions in the room, changing the home base or starting point.

NEGOTIATING CARS AND CAR FAMILIARIZATION

If an older client has difficulty getting into and out of the car due to weakness or stiffness, a vinyl tablecloth or plastic trash bag can be put on the seat to facilitate scooting. Portable handles can be installed in cars to provide stability while entering or exiting (Schwarz, 2008). A swivel car seat—a portable, lightweight cushion with a turntable base—can be used to aid the older adult getting out of the car without putting additional strain on his or her back. (Such products can be obtained from vendors of independent living products for older adults and those with conditions such as arthritis; see the Resources section at the back of this book.)

Stepstools can be provided to help people get into vans. The driver may assist in entering and exiting a van, but the older adult always needs to use caution when using a stepstool. The client's foot should first be placed on the stool without transferring any weight to be sure that the stool is stable. Once the older adult has determined the stool is secure and sturdy, he should locate the roof of the vehicle to avoid hitting his head, and then enter the van. When traveling with a group, it should be announced that the vehicle's doors are closing before doing so to ensure that everyone is out of the way and to prevent possible injury.

To ensure safety when traveling in a car, every passenger should be able to locate these four interior car parts: the interior door handle, the seat belt, the door lock, and the horn. Vehicles today come in so many different configurations that locating all four of these items can sometimes be a challenge. If an accident were to occur or if something were to happen to the driver, older adults with vision loss need to know how to get out of the car or at least blast the horn for assistance.

CANE SKILLS

Using the long white cane to travel independently, without a guide, involves more advanced techniques than the basic skills described so far in this chapter. The O&M instructor considers the need for the long cane and integrates the skills with the older adult's program as well as any technique modifications that may be necessary. Additionally, the O&M instructor takes into account the physical abilities of the older client in determining the type of long cane to be prescribed. Some fundamental information about long cane use and some modifications for older individuals are offered here. Chapter 4 provides a more detailed discussion of the long white cane.

The standard *two-point touch* technique for long white cane use is one of the most basic cane techniques, although the description and instruction may vary slightly by source (Hill & Ponder, 1976; Jacobson, 2013; LaGrow & Long, 2011). The cane is held at midline, extended in front of the body, and moved from side to side, contacting points on the ground just beyond the widest part of the body on the left and the right side, so that the full extent of the terrain in front of the individual's body is covered by the arc of the cane. The cane is raised slightly off the ground as it moves from side to side. The rationale for the technique is discussed in more detail in Chapter 4. The cane tip is supposed to strike the ground opposite the leading (front) foot. That is, the cane tip should touch to the right as the left foot steps down, and the cane tip should touch to the left as the right foot steps down. This is known as "walking in step."

It can be difficult to maintain the cane in the midline position while moving it back and forth. When the midline position is not maintained, protection for both sides of the body is compromised. Using a lighter cane and allowing the arm to be bent slightly at the elbow rather than fully extended allows for a more relaxed position and is easier to maintain. When using this modification, it is important to ensure that the cane covers both sides of the body adequately.

Some older adults may not have the arm strength to use the two-point touch technique appropriately or may have problems with the cane sticking in cracks in the sidewalk or other uneven areas or with the proprioceptive ability to detect drop-offs. A common modification in such instances is to use the *constant-contact* technique and a rolling cane tip rather than the lightweight pencil tip. (Types of cane tips are discussed in more detail in Chapter 4.) When using this technique, the tip of the cane is not lifted off the ground as it moves from side to side, but maintains contact with the walking surface. This constant contact more clearly gives the traveler information about changes in the walking surface as the tip is always touching and small changes are easier to discern. Constant contact not only reduces the amount of wrist movement required but it is better at detecting drop-offs.

An indoor cane technique that is helpful for detecting obstacles is the diagonal technique. In this technique, the cane is held in the dominant hand with the thumb on the flat part of the grip. The grip hand is extended forward approximately 6–8 inches to provide reaction time if objects are contacted. The cane shaft is angled diagonally across the lower part of the body with the tip about 1–2 inches outside the opposite side of the body and elevated

2 inches off the walking surface (Hill & Ponder, 1976; Jacobson, 2013; LaGrow & Long, 2011). However, it may be difficult for the older adult to hold the cane tip off of the floor, and in this position, the elevated tip will not detect surface changes. A modification is the constant contact diagonal, in which the cane tip is in continuous contact with the walking surface. This modification allows detection of surface changes and can be a helpful technique for indoor travel.

SAFETY CONCERNS
Falls

Falling is a serious concern for the older adult population in general, and the chances of falling are increased when there is a visual impairment. When teaching the older adult population it is important to remember that diminished muscle strength and unstable balance are common. Simple exercises can be done to increase arm, leg, and core strength in order to improve balance. More information about falls and fall prevention is provided in Chapter 6.

Solicitation of Aid

Sometimes when older adults are out and about, whether on their own or with a guide, they may find that they are in need of some assistance. It is important for the O&M specialist to encourage older clients to speak up for themselves. Good communication skills are essential under these circumstances. Many older adults who have recently lost vision may be uncomfortable starting conversations. If older adults mention their visual impairment when they first approach someone for assistance or directions, they often find that it is easier to ask that person to identify him- or herself (Griffin-Shirley & Groff, 1993) and to ask for verbal instructions rather than pointing and gestures. For example, someone who has already identified themselves as having a visual impairment might say, "I can't see where you are pointing. Are you suggesting that I go to the right at the corner?" This type of communication can be practiced by role playing different situations to allow older clients to create dialogue appropriate to a variety of scenarios.

Before going to an unfamiliar area, the O&M specialist can have older clients learn as much as possible about the area. Aspects that help with familiarization include the names of streets and businesses near the destination, landmarks, bus stops, and available parking (David, Kollmar, & McCall, 1998,

p. 26). If it becomes necessary to solicit information from someone, the older adult will then have a framework from which to work and any information obtained will, hopefully, be of greater assistance. The O&M specialist can suggest that the older adult ask open-ended questions that require more than "yes" or "no" answers, such as, "What street is this?" or "What is the name of this business?" If the older adult has a hearing loss, encourage him or her to repeat answers in order to verify what was heard, and to ask the person to speak up if necessary. When traveling with a guide, the guide can help to instill confidence in the older adult about orientation and the environment in general. Confidence is important for both travel and personal safety (Bozeman, 2004).

Personal Safety

O&M specialists often concentrate on environmental safety—keeping the instructor and client safe in ever-changing physical surroundings—but another important aspect of O&M instruction is personal safety. Integrating environmental and personal safety is natural for O&M specialists, who often teach backup plans and alternate routes in case the older adult encounters barriers, large crowds, or other impediments to their original plan. These alternate plans can be used for personal safety if the traveler senses an argument or an unsafe situation while traveling. Backup plans that offer concrete alternatives should take into account the amount of time required to escape an unsafe situation and should match the abilities of the client. The amount of time required to escape an unsafe situation would depend on any additional disabilities and physical constraints a client may have. The O&M specialist will want to consider whether the older client can move quickly enough to reverse a given route, or if the identification of periodic safe areas (such as stores or restaurants) would be a better alternative (Bozeman, 2004).

To decrease the chances of becoming the target of a criminal, the older client should exhibit a confident posture and be aware of the environment at all times. Maintaining a confident stride with the head held high also assists with traveling in a straight line and can contribute to improved orientation (Bozeman, 2004).

When moving through a new area, all of the traveler's senses should be engaged to enrich the memory and help with recall. Listening for anything unusual and attending to what types of activities are occurring or smells that are passed may help the older adult remember and be able to retrace his steps.

CHANGING LIVING SITUATIONS

As mental and physical health changes occur, alternative living arrangements and more supportive travel systems (such as alternative travel devices and the use of a human guide) may be required. An older adult who has been living alone using a long white cane may, if his or her health begins to decline, need to learn to use a white cane with a walker or to travel with a guide. Some benefits of a new living environment include support groups and other resources that may become more available as an older individual moves from living alone to living with family members or in a residential facility. The client may be able to go more places and participate in more activities if a new living situation makes more transportation options available.

It is important to find the environment that will provide the best resources to facilitate a safe and comfortable level of independence for each client. Environmental adaptations and modifications are discussed in further detail in Chapters 5 and 7.

SUMMARY

Modifications in traditional O&M skills may need to be made for older adults with visual impairments. Factors such as the person's physical and mental status, living situation, motivation, family support, and transportation access will dictate the type of modifications warranted. The O&M specialist can provide the necessary training with these modifications to assist older adults in maintaining independence in a variety of environments.

LEARNING ACTIVITIES

1. Find an older adult and practice any of the basic O&M skills with modifications required for the older adult discussed in this chapter. Get feedback from the older adult about the activity.
2. Simulate sensory loss and age-related physical impairment by doing the following:
    a. Use ear plugs to simulate a hearing loss.
    b. Put gloves on and tape your thumb and index finger together on your dominant hand to simulate the neuropathy and loss of dexterity.
    c. Tape a paint stirrer to both sides of your knee to stiffen it to simulate decreased range of motion.

d. Put on a blindfold and trail the length of a hallway. (Be sure to have a spotter for this simulation activity.) Reflect on the experience.
3. Practice getting in and out of chairs and cars with the methods described in this chapter.
4. Read the Appendix, "O&M for Older Individuals with Visual Impairment in Rural Areas: Reflections from an O&M Specialist in Alaska." Write a reflection paper on how you personally use weather, topography, and climatology to assist your orientation in various environments.

References

Benson, S. (n.d.). *So what about independent travel?* Baltimore: National Federation of the Blind. Retrieved from https://nfb.org/images/nfb/documents/pdf/article_sowhataboutindependenttravel_lbs05p.pdf

Bentzen, B. L., & Marston, J. R. (2010). Teaching the use of orientation aids for orientation and mobility. In W. R. Wiener, R. L. Welsh, & B. B. Blasch (Eds.), *Foundations of orientation and mobility: Vol. II. Instructional strategies and practical applications* (3rd ed., pp. 315–351). New York: AFB Press.

Bozeman, L. A. (2004). Environmental and personal safety: No vision required [Practice report]. *Journal of Visual Impairment & Blindness, 98*(7), 434–438.

Bozeman, L. A., & McCulley, R. M. (2010). Improving orientation for students with vision loss. In W. R. Wiener, R. L. Welsh, & B. B. Blasch (Eds.), *Foundations of orientation and mobility: Vol. II. Instructional strategies and practical applications* (3rd ed., pp. 27–53). New York: AFB Press.

Carleyy. (n.d.). 25 unique uses for pantyhose (step 4). *Instructables.* Retrieved from http://www.instructables.com/id/25-Unique-Uses-for-Pantyhose

David, W., Kollmar, K., & McCall, S. (1998). *Safe without sight: Crime prevention and self-defense strategies for people who are blind.* Boston: National Braille Press.

Gallagher, W. F. (1974). The elbow has an intelligence quotient. *The New Outlook for the Blind, 68.*

Griffin-Shirley, N., & Groff, G. (1993). *Prescriptions for independence: Working with older people who are visually impaired.* New York: AFB Press.

Griffin-Shirley, N., & Welsh, R. L. (2010). Teaching orientation and mobility to older adults. In W. R. Wiener, R. L. Welsh, & B. B. Blasch (Eds.), *Foundations of orientation and mobility: Vol. II. Instructional strategies and practical applications* (3rd ed., pp. 286–311). New York: AFB Press.

Hill, E., & Ponder, P. (1976). *Orientation and mobility techniques: A guide for the practitioner.* New York: American Foundation for the Blind.

Jacobson, W. H. (2013). *The art and science of teaching orientation and mobility to persons with visual impairments* (2nd ed.). New York: AFB Press.

LaGrow, S. J., & Long, R. G. (2011). *Orientation and mobility: Techniques for independence* (2nd ed.). Alexandria, VA: Association for Education and Rehabilitation of the Blind and Visually Impaired.

National Osteoporosis Foundation. (n.d.). *Proper body alignment*. Washington, DC: Author. Retrieved from http://nof.org/articles/549

Pogrund, R., Sewell, D., Anderson, H., Calaci, L., Cowart, M. F., Gonzalez, C. M., . . . Roberson-Smith, B. (2012). Part 3: Appendices. In *Teaching age-appropriate purposeful skills (TAPS): An orientation and mobility curriculum for students with visual impairments* (3rd ed.). Austin: Texas School for the Blind and Visually Impaired.

Rosen, S., & Crawford, J. S. (2010). Teaching orientation and mobility to learners with visual, physical, and health impairments. In W. R. Wiener, R. L. Welsh, & B. B. Blasch (Eds.), *Foundations of orientation and mobility: Vol. II. Instructional strategies and practical applications* (3rd ed., pp. 564–623). New York: AFB Press.

Rushforth, A. (2009). *Suggestions for teaching: Positioning the arm for self-protective techniques*. Unpublished manuscript, Lander, WY.

Schwarz, S. P. (2008, April). Getting in and out of cars. *Mobility Corner*. Retrieved from http://www.mobilitycorner.com/getting-in-and-out.html

Welsh, R. L. (2010). Improving psychosocial functioning for orientation and mobility. In W. R. Wiener, R. L. Welsh, & B. B. Blasch (Eds.), *Foundations of orientation and mobility: Vol. II. Instructional strategies and practical applications* (3rd ed., pp. 138–159). New York: AFB Press.

APPENDIX 3A
O&M for Older Individuals with Visual Impairment in Rural Areas
Reflections from an O&M Specialist in Alaska

John Clare

Though my teaching experience has primarily taken place in a rural area of Alaska, the information in this section can be applied to any population of older adults with visual impairments, whether they live out in the country or in the middle of a large city.

An O&M specialist working with a population of older people in a rural area must be able to do three things:

1. Understand the needs of the population.
2. Coordinate his or her work with clients and their significant others within the community.
3. Understand how local geography and climate affect a client's ability to be oriented in space.

The O&M specialist working in a rural community will need to learn some of the psychosocial aspects of rural populations and to become an amateur geographer and climatologist.

UNDERSTANDING THE NEEDS OF OLDER ADULTS WITH VISUAL IMPAIRMENTS AND OTHERS IN A RURAL COMMUNITY

Understanding what life is like in rural areas means understanding how rural areas make unique demands on those who live there. Questions to consider about a client in a rural area include the following:

- Is the client active in the community?
- If not, is he or she uninvolved by choice?

- Does the client have friends or family members who provide steady companionship?

Rural communities, like many close-knit communities, often have a sense that they are unique and that they possess values and traditions that must be protected. Small communities, bound together by common need, often do an excellent job of caring for their older neighbors and family. Providing assistance to individuals who live in small communities consequently requires extra tact and insight. Rural people often perceive people from the "outside" as irritating, nosey, and unsophisticated. Indeed, too often the impression that the well-intentioned and sometimes insensitive outsider leaves is more negative than positive. It is critical, therefore, that the O&M specialist enter a small community carefully, with humility, and with the goal of making a good first impression. A great way to make an immediate, positive impression is to be a good listener, as the experiences described here will illustrate.

My clients in rural Alaska generally fall into two categories: those who are an integral part of their community and those who, often by choice, live a relatively isolated existence.

The Older Individual Living as Part of a Community

There are approximately 230 villages in Alaska. The majority of them are accessible only by airplane or boat. For geographical and logistical reasons, Alaskan village infrastructure also tends to be very compact, with buildings and houses situated very close to one another. Alaskan villages, not unlike rural communities anywhere in the world, are typically populated by people who have lived shoulder to shoulder for many generations. This situation—geographical remoteness paired with close community living—requires that residents develop a tremendously sophisticated set of communication skills in order to coexist and survive.

The city dweller having a bad day may take his or her frustration out on a clerk at the supermarket, knowing that there is another market close by should the behavior alienate the shopkeeper. That same behavior, exhibited in a small rural community, may very well mean that the grumpy shopper must have his or her batch of groceries flown in from another supplier!

Rural, older adults who are visually impaired frequently have their activities and daily living needs met—as a matter of course, and as a point of pride—by their extended families, their neighbors, or both. Very often, people in small communities do not think of their older adults with visual impairments as disabled. How can they be disabled if all their needs are met?

Within this culture, if an O&M specialist arrives in a small community and, without family input, proposes to teach an older adult to become independent in his or her daily activities, this may be perceived as a threat. Even if the older adult desires more independence, the specialist may unwittingly jeopardize the individual's standing within the family and community by asking him or her to choose between that desired independence and harmony with others.

Rural societies often hold older adults in high regard. Indigenous rural Alaskans typically refer to their older citizens as Elders. In these communities, growing old confers a high degree of respect. Older adults in rural Alaska are often valued for their ability to pass on oral traditions and teach important life skills. It is critical, then, for the O&M specialist to do some homework on the community or communities he or she serves, and to take the time to build good relationships with the families and caregivers that are active in his or her clients' lives. A good rapport with the villagers is the gateway to teaching older adults with visual impairments.

Albert's Story

> A number of years ago, when I was contracting with an independent living center in Fairbanks to provide O&M services to older adults with vision loss in Alaska's interior, people would occasionally drop by and suggest visiting an elderly man living in a small village of about 150 residents that I'll call Hannah Creek. After deciding to learn what I could about the man, my first step was to call Barbara, the Hannah Creek Village Health Aide. Almost every village in Alaska has a health aide. They are typically local women trained by the Indian Health Service to provide minor medical assistance to local residents. For obvious reasons, health aides are normally the ones "in the know" about their communities. I knew that to be an effective service provider to this man, I would need to have Barbara on my side.
>
> I asked Barbara if an older man who was blind and might need help lived in the village. The response was a quick "No." By her terse reply it was obvious that getting on Barbara's good side was not going to be easy. I rephrased the question, asking if there was a man who was blind in the village, but leaving out the part about needing help. Again her answer was "No." I didn't want to be a nuisance, so I thanked her and ended the phone call. The following month, I called Barbara again. After talking about the

weather and the past fishing season, I asked if a man who was blind lived in Hannah Creek. Her answer was, "No." I thanked her, told her we would talk again someday, and ended the call. The next month, I called again. After the obligatory weather and fishing conversation, I asked if there were an older man living in Hannah Creek who didn't see very well. After a long pause she replied, "Maybe." Sensing that we might be getting somewhere, I asked: "Barbara, if I happen to stop by Hannah Creek while on my way to another village, may I come introduce myself to you?" She told me that this would be possible. When I asked if I could pick up anything for her or the clinic at the store in Fairbanks, I could tell she appreciated the offer.

A month or two later I had the opportunity to go to Hannah Creek and meet Barbara. After finding the village clinic, I had a chance to sit down with her and get to know each other a bit. To begin with, she accepted some inexpensive low vision items that she could give to the local people: easy-to-thread needles, a few 20/20 pens, and some check and signature writing guides. We talked about common forms of visual impairment and a few techniques for screening people for vision problems. Eventually Barbara said, "There is an old man here, his name is Albert, and he is blind, but he is not disabled." I considered what she said before asking her what she meant by "not disabled." She replied, "Disabled people need help, but Albert has everything he needs. He has his family and neighbors."

That afternoon Barbara introduced me to Albert and his family at Albert's house. Albert was in his 80s, had retinitis pigmentosa and profound hearing loss, and did not speak English. I spent most of the afternoon teaching the family guiding techniques and some very simple constant contact cane techniques. I gave Albert a long white cane with a large, bright red roller ball tip, and he gave me a big smile.

This story shows how important it is for O&M specialists to build relationships and trust with the caregivers in their clients' communities. The more isolated the community is linguistically, geographically, and culturally, the more important these relationships usually become.

It is also important for the O&M specialist to understand that the concept of independence is a fluid one that will vary from client to client and community to community. Had I compared Albert's O&M skills to those of clients who had had more training, I could have come to the conclusion that Albert's family simply enabled his helplessness. In fact, in his later years, Albert's family and community depended on him to enrich their lives. The relationships were interdependent. Barbara was right: Albert was not disabled.

It is also important for the O&M specialist to demonstrate discretion, to keep the private details of clients' lives and the lives of their families confidential. By refraining from any form of gossip during the first meeting, I convinced Barbara that her own hard-won reputation in the community would not be challenged by my presence.

O&M specialists will have the best chance at success if they strive to meet the immediate needs of their clients, even if a given skill doesn't fall into the correct scope and sequence of typical O&M training. Albert liked to walk outdoors by himself once in a while and to sit and smoke his pipe. To do this, he had to travel up and down a long set of stairs, which worried his family. Because of this immediate need, I prioritized teaching Albert the proper cane technique for stair travel, even though that particular cane skill is normally considered somewhat advanced.

O&M specialists in rural communities ought to take any opportunity they find to share their expertise with others. In the village of Hannah Creek, I took the time to connect a portable video magnifier (also called closed-circuit television system or CCTV) to the senior center's enormous television. When people saw what the magnifier could do, a group of six older women—who had just 10 minutes earlier been perturbed because I'd interrupted their favorite afternoon TV program—silently got up from their chairs, went to their rooms, and came back with their Bibles and beadwork to put under the video magnifier's camera lens!

The Older Individual Living in an Isolated Setting

There are older individuals in all parts of the country who—either by choice or turn of events—live alone. Even if they choose isolation, such individuals often may have difficulty living independently with confidence. Interestingly, the needs of these isolated individuals are in many ways the same whether they live in the middle of a large city or 50 miles from their nearest neighbor. O&M specialists may become part of a team of people charged with helping these individuals or may find themselves functioning as the initial contact, responsible in part for connecting the older adult with others who can assist.

Alaska has its share of recluses. More often than not, these individuals are older men who, for reasons unknown, do not enjoy the company of close neighbors. This situation can be a challenge because reconnection with society may need to be part of their O&M training. Respect for the life choices of such individuals is the key to having any influence on their lives.

Turk's Story

The referral for Turk came from a public health nurse who was concerned about his safety in and around his home. Turk lived on a quiet stretch of river not far from neighbors but perhaps 20 miles from the nearest small town. He moved to his cabin years before in order to enjoy retirement on the edge of a fine little salmon river. In his 70s, not long after Turk moved to the river, he developed the wet form of macular degeneration. Within a year, he had lost most of the central vision in both eyes. To make matters worse, he was also diagnosed with terminal cancer. This was quite a blow for someone who had been a fighter pilot in World War II. His passion was tying salmon flies and seeing what he could catch with them.

After we shared a cup of coffee, Turk announced that he was just fine and that he would not need O&M instruction or help. "Everyone wants me to move to town but I'm not going so you may as well hit the road," he stated matter-of-factly. I decided to ignore his comment for the time being and instead asked about a photo on the wall: "I'm a pilot—can you tell me about the guy standing on the wing of that Corsair?" For the next hour, he told one story after another from his years as a young World War II naval aviator who fought in the South Pacific.

Over the next year, I came to Turk's place once a month. He learned about video magnifiers, talking books, and O&M. We ended each visit with a cup of coffee and endless stories. Turk never did leave his place. He was a proud and independent man who, with the assistance of some understanding people, managed to live on his own to the end.

I've found that the key to convincing a reluctant individual to accept the skills we have to teach as O&M professionals and put them into practice is to show him or her that I care. There is no better way to do this than by finding common ground through shared experiences. For example, when Turk found out that I was also a pilot, he knew that I would understand something important about him.

The life choices of others are worthy of respect, no matter how different they may be from our own. When Turk insisted that he was fine right where he was and suggested that I hit the road, it was evident that he saw me as one in a long line of people who had been attempting to persuade him to move closer to town. As soon as the opportunity in the conversation appeared, I let him know that I respected his choice to live where he wanted to.

Turk's story also demonstrates the importance of perseverance. When a client is reluctant to receive O&M services, the best course of action for the O&M specialist may be to let it go, then call back in a month to see if a short appointment can be arranged.

Many seniors (and Turk was one of these) like clear, direct instruction. Telling the client exactly what is planned for the day, teaching the skill explicitly, and recapping the lesson can all contribute to fostering mutual respect between a specialist and the client. Older adults frequently hold the teaching profession in high regard and they appreciate a businesslike approach to instruction.

O&M specialists are in some ways salespeople. Convincing a client or family member to take a risk or try something new will depend not just on the client's trust in the specialist, but in the specialist's skills in persuasion and his or her ability to deliver on promises.

UNDERSTANDING HOW GEOGRAPHY AND LOCAL WEATHER AFFECT NAVIGATION

For thousands of years, humans have completed amazing feats of navigation, traveling through jungles, forests, and deserts with little more than the wind, sun, and stars as aids. Instructors may use weather and topography to aid in their O&M training. Today, O&M instructors teach sophisticated cane techniques along with how to combine those techniques with all kinds of micro clues and landmarks. But what about the larger geographic and atmospheric environment—the macro environment, so to speak? In a rural area in particular, paying attention to the land and the climate, and how it affects the life of the community, is crucial.

Weather patterns are just that, patterns. O&M specialists need to understand how weather affects the communities in which they teach and make sure that their clients understand local weather patterns. Talking to old timers, along with working and playing outside, can give the O&M specialist insight into how weather affects a given rural community.

For the rural O&M client, understanding cardinal or compass directions can be critical. Imagine a traveler who is blind walking down a long dirt road that runs north-south. She walks down the road to the mailbox, but on the way home she becomes disoriented. She knows that her mailbox is south of her home and that her home is two miles inland from the Pacific Ocean. It is early afternoon and a hard onshore breeze is blowing from the west. If she has an understanding of compass directions, she would know that if she puts the breeze on her left shoulder, then she will be pointed north to walk home.

A number of years ago, I had a memorable older client who was blind who went by the nickname Porky. Porky, another World War II Navy veteran, spent his life at sea as a Navy man. Porky's career at sea and his lifelong interest in hunting and the outdoors provided him with an exceptional ability to be well orientated, a hard-won skill of which he is particularly proud. Occasionally, though, Porky could become disoriented and when that happened, he would show another trait common to exceptional travelers, the ability to remain in place. Porky would stop, lean on his cane, close his eyes, and lower his head, sometimes for up to five or more minutes. Any attempt to talk to him was a waste of time; he was lost in thought. Eventually, Porky would calmly lift his head, grab his cane, turn in the proper direction, and start walking. Eventually, he explained this technique. Porky explained his technique this way: "I used to smoke a pipe, and that's when I seemed to do most of my productive thinking. Now, just as soon as I realize I am lost, I stop and picture myself sitting on a log, smoking that old pipe. Then, I just calmly and logically think about where I might be and where I need to go and it comes to me!" When disoriented, Porky was able to remain calm to deduce the correct direction.

The people of Alaska are dependent on the extraction of natural resources for many cultural and economic reasons. Access to natural resources tends to be seasonal by nature. People must pay special attention to the local climate and geography because their lives and livelihoods are at stake. It has been my experience that, with few exceptions, older adults who have lived much of their lives outdoors are very well oriented. They know where north is, where the mountains are, where the ocean is, and they know most every geographic feature necessary for cross-country travel.

HOWARD'S STORY

Finally, as O&M specialists, it is worthwhile to consider the unique balancing act that some of our clients must perform within their communities. Travelers must be aware of other's concerns about their safety and at the same time work to prove they can be independent travelers. Sometimes this is an easy process, sometimes it is difficult, and sometimes it can be humorous.

Howard, a client and friend of mine, called me soon after he and his wife Marie moved to the small Athabascan community of Fort Yukon on the banks of the upper Yukon River. Both Howard, who has been blind since birth, and Marie, who is sighted, love to run. At the time he called, they often ran as a pair, holding on to the same short rope. Marie ran in the lead with Howard right behind. When he called, Howard laughed and said, "I need you to come teach me how to get around this village, man—people are talking." "What do you mean by 'talking'?" I asked. "Well," Howard said, "the other evening Marie and I went for a run. We had a good run, but the next morning several village elders knocked on our door. They told me that they didn't like the way Marie was treating me. I told them I didn't know what they were talking about, and they replied, "We saw your wife pulling you all over the place with a rope last night and we don't think that's right!"

Howard wanted to learn a route from his house to the store and post office so he could demonstrate to his new neighbors that he could travel independently just fine. I flew out to Fort Yukon. Howard began his route familiarization and instruction by walking to the store from his house. As we headed down the dirt road, which was full of potholes, one of Howard's neighbors came out of his house and walked quickly to intercept us. He did not look happy. The man blocked our way, then turned and stood to face me. In a low and threatening voice he said, "This is my friend, Howard. I am going to watch you every minute to make sure nothing bad happens to him!" Then he turned and walked back into his house. Howard laughed and said "Man, a guy can't get away with anything around here!"

In just a few days, Howard, a gifted traveler, learned the new route using all of the clues and landmarks typical of a rural Alaskan community. These clues included the sound of the generator rumbling behind the store, the sound of a halyard banging in the wind on the aluminum post office flagpole, and the sound of hungry dog teams staked out around the village. Howard was able to demonstrate to the villagers that he was just another person, that he was independent in his travel, and that he could live safely in the community. Come to think of it, though, he never said if he and Marie continued to run together using a rope.

These anecdotes demonstrate only some of the challenges and benefits of working in rural communities. I'd like to leave my fellow O&M specialists with the following advice:

- Take the time to get to know your clients and the people in their communities.
- Give your clients respect and they will learn to trust you and work to put into practice the skills that you have taught.
- Take time to learn salient information about the local geography and climate.
- Identify and validate each client's present level of understanding and then build on that base.
- Encourage each client to believe that everyone is capable of learning to become a better traveler.

CHAPTER 4

Orientation and Mobility Tools and Techniques

James Scott Crawford

A wide variety of tools are available to assist people with visual impairments with their mobility needs. These tools can be divided into three categories: devices that assist with probing the environment (such as the long white cane), devices that assist with support or balance, and devices that assist with maintaining orientation (Smith & Penrod, 2010).

Many older adults with vision loss utilize more than one type of device and some may use multiple devices at the same time. An older adult's choice of device may vary based on type of trip, length of trip, time of day, environment to be traveled, familiarity with the area, fluctuating vision and health, and the level of assistance available from others. A client may choose to use a support cane for one trip, but select a wheelchair for a longer trip. Clients' physical, visual, and cognitive abilities vary and should be taken into consideration when determining what tools to utilize and when. Older adults may choose to use a long cane only at night or in unfamiliar environments. It is important for orientation and mobility (O&M) specialists to prepare clients for the wide variety of situations they will encounter in their daily lives and to familiarize them with the range of options that are available to meet their O&M needs. Sources for many of the products discussed in this chapter can be found in the Resources section at the end of this book.

CONSULTATION WITH OTHER PROFESSIONALS

O&M specialists are part of a rehabilitation team that consists of other professionals such as physical therapists and physicians. For an older adult with disabilities in addition to vision loss, some standard interventions may cause pain or injury, or cause him or her to be unsafe. By collaborating with team members, O&M specialists can help ensure that the techniques and strategies used are those that best meet the client's needs. (See Sidebar 1.3 for a discussion of team members and Chapter 8 for strategies for effective collaboration.)

LONG WHITE CANES

The use of the long white cane for independent travel and specific cane techniques was introduced in Chapter 3. The long white cane is used as a probe to investigate the environment as the individual travels, clear the path ahead of obstacles, check for drop-offs, or follow a wall or other shoreline. Support canes are discussed later in this chapter.

Types of White Canes

Long white canes can be made of just about any available material, but most often are made of aluminum, carbon fiber, or fiberglass. Older adults with visual impairments often own more than one cane. They may prefer one type for indoor use and a different type for outdoor use, or one type for trips in vehicles and a different type for walking substantial distances. Some older adults will use one type of cane during the day and a different type at night when their vision is less reliable (Geruschat & Smith, 2010).

The length of the cane depends on the client's stride length, speed, and reaction time. O&M specialists issue canes ranging in height from anywhere between the height of the client's sternum to the height of his or her forehead. In theory, the cane should be long enough that the tip lands in the spot where the next foot moving forward would land. In reality, the cane needs to sweep wide enough to clear a path at least as wide as the older adult's body and extend far enough forward that the older adult has time to react when the cane encounters an obstacle. Since foot placement is generally narrower than the body's width, this means that the cane tip should hit to the side of where the foot will land. With the hand grasping the cane in a natural position, and the client walking at his or her fastest pace, the footfall should not land beyond where the most recent cane tip has landed. In other words, if the next footfall lands beyond the point last hit by the cane, the cane is too short. For many people, the amount of forward arm extension decreases when training does not focus on cane skills. This reduces the amount of forward reach, which creates a need for a longer cane. O&M specialists who assume older adults will always keep their cane arms fully extended may issue canes that are too short to maintain safety (Crawford & Crawford, in press).

Canes can be rigid, folding, or telescoping. The vibrotactile information (the perception of vibration through touch) relayed by a rigid cane is the most accurate of the three types, as it is not distorted by the vibrations that can occur at the joints of folding and telescoping canes. The absence of joints allows rigid canes to be thinner and lighter. Rigid canes are also stronger and less likely to break. However, they do not have the advantage of a folding cane, which is more convenient to store when traveling in vehicles or when seated.

Telescoping canes are compact when collapsed, very lightweight, and provide better vibrotactile information than folding canes. The disadvantage is that telescoping canes tend to collapse when needed most, such as when the tip gets caught in a crack while in the middle of a street crossing. Many older adults request folding canes because they are easier to stow in vehicles or when out and about, and they can be put in a pocket or purse when not needed.

No matter what type of cane a client uses, the best cane in the world does no good sitting in a closet. Some older adults, especially those with usable vision, tend to leave their canes at home instead of using them. It is the role of O&M specialists to help their older clients learn when canes are necessary and when they can be set aside. O&M specialists should help their older clients understand that although a cane may not seem necessary when they walk out the door, once they are on their way, circumstances may change and they may find they need a cane after all.

Cane Tips

All canes come with tips that can be replaced when they wear out. The type of tip an older adult prefers will depend on the cane technique he or she uses most often. Older adults may prefer one type of cane tip for indoor use and a different tip for outdoor use (Smith & Penrod, 2010). See Figure 4.1 for different types of cane tips.

Pencil tips are short, narrow tips, usually 1–2 inches long and roughly the same diameter as the shaft of the cane. They are lightweight and relatively long-lasting and are excellent for use with the two-point touch technique. They provide good auditory and vibrotactile feedback. However, pencil tips tend to get stuck easily in cracks in the sidewalk or other uneven surfaces when used in the constant-contact technique, in which the tip of the cane remains in contact with the walking surface and the traveler is walking in-step (Jacobson, 2013). (Walking in-step means the cane tip strikes the ground opposite the leading or front foot. See Chapter 3 for additional description of cane techniques.)

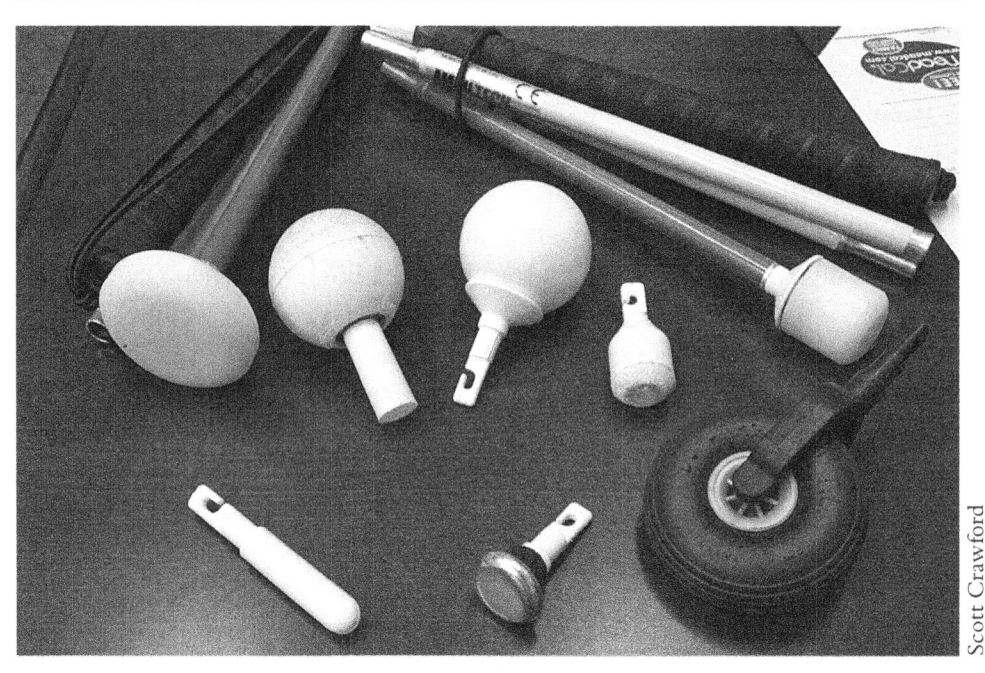

FIGURE **4.1**
A wide variety of cane tips are available to travelers who are visually impaired including pencil, marshmallow/mushroom, metal glide, roller, roller ball, jumbo roller, wheel, and all-terrain.

Marshmallow tips and *mushroom caps* are round tips that are heavier and larger than pencil tips, measuring an inch or more in diameter. They are often used with the constant-contact technique. These types of tips are less likely than pencil tips to get stuck in cracks or grass.

Metal glide tips are flat, round tips that produce the clearest auditory and vibrotactile information (Crawford & Crawford, in press). These tips are fairly durable when used with the two-point touch technique, but wear out quickly when used outdoors with the constant-contact technique. Metal glide tips are traditionally used on canes made of fiberglass, such as the cane made by the National Federation of the Blind (NFB), but are also available for use with aluminum or carbon fiber folding or rigid canes.

Roller tips are designed for use with the constant-contact technique. These tips, which have a small wheel at the end, are approximately the size of a large marshmallow. Roller tips do not get stuck as frequently as non-rolling tips. However, when roller tips are used with the two-point touch technique, the cane can seem very heavy. Roller tips are long-lasting even when used with the constant-contact technique. If the older client tends to push the cane in a straight line instead of keeping the tip rolling, one side of the tip will wear faster than the other sides. The tip will develop a flat section that will either prevent the tip from rolling or will cause a thumping vibration that may lead to the client missing important tactile information. As a roller tip ages, the bearings inside the wheel may become noisy, which can mask auditory information.

Roller ball tips are similar to roller tips, but instead of a wheel, their rolling mechanism is the size and shape of a billiard ball. They are made of a less durable, lighter weight material than roller tips, and thus they tend to wear out faster. Roller ball tips usually skip out of smaller cracks that cause other tips to stick. Roller ball tips perform well in grass. These tips are usually preferred by people who move at a quick pace and who mainly use the constant-contact technique (Crawford & Crawford, in press).

Jumbo roller tips are shaped like a donut. These tips are made of heavy nylon, which makes them durable but very heavy. Fast walkers may find that the jumbo roller tips have a tendency to skip, jump, and bounce along the sidewalk, while slower walkers will find that they roll smoothly. When installed on a long cane, the jumbo roller tip can provide a small amount of support at curbs and on stairs. To provide support, it is vital that the cane be held straight up and down so the tip does not roll. If the cane is held at an angle, the tip can roll, so it will not provide support.

Wheel tips are primarily used by people who cannot lift their cane. They are frequently used with the diagonal technique, in which the cane is held at an angle in front of the individual and not swung side to side. In order to move the cane side to side, the older adult must be able to perform a radial-ulnar twist (the same movement as turning a door knob), changing the angle at which the wheel is contacting the ground and allowing it to roll across the older adult's path.

All-terrain tips take the form of skids or runners that curve forward from the shaft of the cane. They are used on dirt, gravel, and grass surfaces. The tip design allows the user to slide it over rough surfaces without getting stuck.

Cane Grips

For people who have problems grasping the cane, the type of grip can be important. NFB-style canes tend to have hard plastic handles that are thinner than other types of cane handles. Because the shafts of NFB canes are usually made of fiberglass or carbon fiber, they can be thinner than canes made of other materials. Some older clients may find it easier to hold these thinner canes. However, the thinner handle may cause problems for people who have hand pain or who struggle to close their fingers. The *golf grips* used on aluminum and some carbon fiber canes are usually made of rubber and are softer, larger, and heavier than NFB-style cane handles. Handles and grips can be built up by adding cloth tape, leather tape (as used on tennis racquet grips), or pipe insulation. Increasing the diameter of a grip may make the cane easier to hold, but additional layers may cause a loss of sensitivity to the tactile feedback from the cane. Physical and occupational therapists are good sources for grip materials.

The following is an example of a situation in which adapting the long white cane can be helpful to an older adult with a visual impairment:

> George has severe neuropathy and is unable to feel surface changes or drop-offs with his cane. To increase the sound cues from his cane, George placed several large washers on the shaft, just above the tip. After he made this adaptation, when George's cane tip hit uneven surfaces or went over a drop-off, the "chank-chank" sound of the washers alerted him to the uneven footing.

Adaptive Mobility Devices

There are a wide variety of adaptive mobility devices (AMDs) that are designed to clear the travel path for individuals who either cannot swing a cane or who have not yet learned to use a cane safely. Some AMDs are homemade devices created for an individual user, while other AMDs are available commercially. Most AMDs are generally rectangular in shape and are made out of aluminum or PVC piping (see Figure 4.2). A traveler usually pushes an AMD in front of him- or herself; AMDs are not usually swept side to side. Older clients may hold on to the top of an AMD, like pushing a shopping cart. When used as a transition to cane use, the devices can also be pushed by the sides or by handles, which can put the hands in a position similar to that used for the long white cane.

Depending on the design, the AMDs may have supports, wheels, or tips that will indicate drop-offs to the front and, sometimes, sides of the client. With devices that slide or roll on a horizontal bar, older adults may not detect the edge of the sidewalk because the center of the bar may be supported by that edge and the client does not have the perception of a "drop."

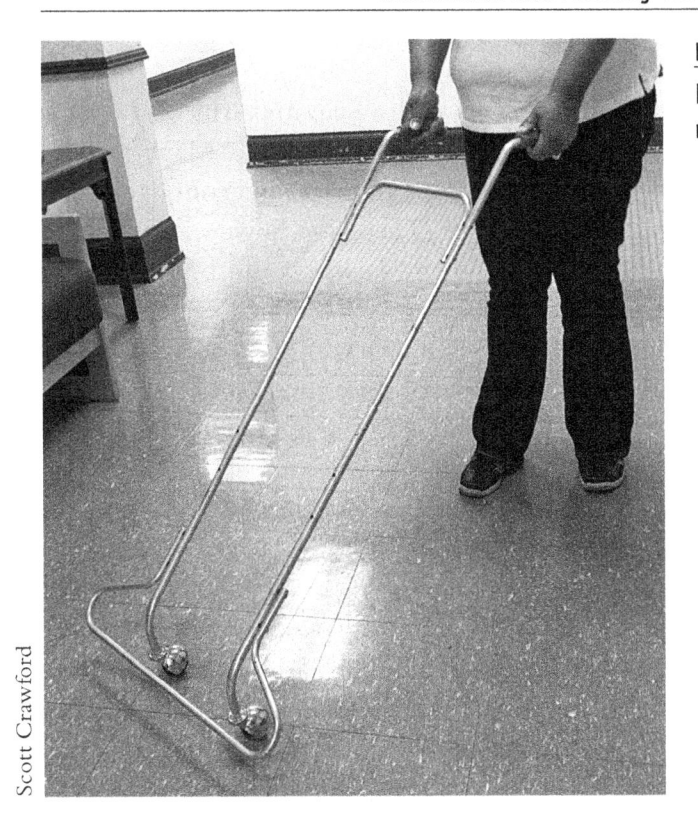

FIGURE **4.2**

Example of an adaptive mobility device.

Cane Alternatives

Until they receive formal O&M training, many people who are visually impaired use nontraditional alternatives to the long cane—such as fishing poles, pool cues, car antennas, curtain rods, brooms, walking sticks, tree branches, or any other long, thin object—to help them get around. Before discarding these types of objects, O&M specialists will want to consider why the individual may have picked a particular cane alternative and what advantages that object may offer over traditional canes. A person using a walking stick or other heavy object may be looking for support as well as a probe for the environment. For example, one individual utilized a broom to probe the sidewalk; when there was loose gravel, leaves, or twigs, she used the broom to sweep the path for herself. She also leaned on the broom when she needed to rest. Observing this provided the O&M specialist with evidence of stamina issues, balance issues, and discomfort with uneven or loose footing (Crawford & Crawford, in press).

DOG GUIDES

Dog guides are typically utilized by people with visual impairments over the age of 16. The decision to use a dog guide is a personal one. Many users of dog guides find that the dog provides a sense of freedom and confidence that they do not feel when traveling with a cane. There are, however, minimum physical requirements for dog guide handlers, such as a minimum level of hearing and a maximum amount of vision, as well as added responsibilities that come with using dog guides. In addition to having to feed and care for the dog, the dog's handler must be committed to traveling on a regular basis, since regular practice is necessary for both the dog and the user to retain their training and physical health. For specific requirements and expectations, the older client should be referred to the school to which he or she is planning to apply (Franck, Haneline, Brooks, & Whitstock, 2010).

For many people, the advantages of having a dog guide them around obstacles and hazards make up for not being able to explore everything in the environment with a cane. Dog guide users must be able to maintain their orientation based on what they hear, what they feel under foot, and the information received through the dog's harness. Some schools have started allowing older adults to simultaneously use a dog guide and a cane, electronic travel aids, or global positioning systems (GPS) to assist with maintaining orientation, determining position, and finding landmarks (Franck et al., 2010).

ORTHOPEDIC EQUIPMENT

As noted at the beginning of the chapter, it is crucial for the O&M specialist working with an older adult to consult with other specialists on the individual's rehabilitation team to make sure the client's needs don't fall through the cracks among specialties. Older clients who are visually impaired often have additional orthopedic impairments that the O&M specialist will want to take into consideration before beginning training. Under these circumstances, consultations with physical therapists and occupational therapists are vital to gain a complete understanding of the best approach to ensure safety while maximizing independence. O&M specialists should always defer to the guidance of these team members when it comes to recommending devices and measurement and setting up equipment. That being said, older adults often possess equipment that has not been recommended, set up, or adjusted by an appropriate professional. O&M specialists should familiarize themselves with the standard settings for orthopedic equipment and encourage their clients to ask for assistance from their occupational and physical therapists with getting the appropriate types and sizes of equipment. O&M specialists need to keep in mind that the safety and effectiveness of any technique depends on the older client's individual strengths, weaknesses, and skill level.

Support Canes

Support canes can help redistribute weight for lower extremity pain or weakness and can improve stability by increasing the base of support. They are available in a wide variety of shapes, sizes, materials, colors, lengths, and tip types. While some people will need a support cane to prevent falls, others may need support when they stumble or when they walk on uneven surfaces or slopes. In some cases, the support cane may be needed only for ascending or descending curbs and stairs. Many people use a white support cane as a form of identification as a person with a visual impairment, or as a fashion statement. Some people may carry support canes without really knowing why.

White support canes are intended to indicate that the person using it has a visual impairment. White tape can be added to a cane that is a different color. For the client's safety, a physician, physical therapist, or occupational therapist should specify the length and tip type of a support cane (Rosen & Crawford, 2010). However, support canes are often acquired without the assistance of medical professionals. Many are inherited from relatives and may be inappropriate for the person using them. Others are purchased at garage sales or drug stores and are never fitted to the user. For an insurance company to pay for a support cane, a physician's prescription is usually required.

The optimum length of a support cane varies based on the height of the user, the length of the user's arm, the strategy for use of the cane, and the positioning of the cane while walking. As a general rule for someone using a support cane, the top of the handle should be the same height from the ground as the user's wristbone when his or her hand is dangling freely at the side of his or her body. While some older adults may prefer a longer cane, a support cane of this length is usually most comfortable for walking with weight being supported by the cane. If the cane is too long, the older adult's shoulder may be pushed up uncomfortably, or the cane and arm may not stay aligned, which can lead to weaker support from the cane. If the older adult who is visually impaired uses the cane as a probe, it may need to be longer than normal. This will lead to less support, but the cane can then be used to clear the path ahead, check for drop-offs, or follow a wall or other shoreline (border of the area being walked through).

It is beyond the scope of an O&M specialist to recommend that an older client stop using a support cane or to change how the client uses the support cane. If, however, an O&M specialist is concerned that an older client is not using the support cane properly, or that the client may need a different amount of support, attempts should be made to consult with the client's physician, physical therapist, or occupational therapist. While it is commonly said that the support cane should be used on the side opposite the weaker leg, in fact, the side of use depends on the location and type of weakness. The physician, physical therapist, or occupational therapist should determine on which side the support cane should be positioned (Rosen & Crawford, 2010).

Support canes can come with a variety of tips and bases. Some can be used in either hand, while others are designed to be used on a specific side of the body. Metal-tipped canes should have a rubber cap in place over the metal tip. The purpose of the metal is to keep the cane from wearing down or splitting, but metal tips are very slick and provide no reliable support. The rubber tip allows the cane to stay in position on the floor. If the rubber tip wears unevenly, it should be replaced. If the metal under the rubber tip becomes exposed, it can lead to the tip slipping (Rosen & Crawford, 2010).

Quad canes (which have four legs) and tripod canes (which have three legs) offer a wider base and greater stability than standard canes. These models have legs that are arranged off-center from the shaft of the cane. The cane shaft attaches to the base closer to two of the legs, with the other side of the base extending farther out from the shaft (see Figure 4.3A). The cane should be held so that the side closer to the shaft is next to the older adult's body. If held in the wrong position, the cane will provide less support and will become a tripping hazard for the user (see Figure 4.3B). If for some reason the older adult must hold the cane in the hand opposite of the one intended by the cane's design, the handle of the cane can be turned around backward so the base still extends away from the user's feet (Rosen & Crawford, 2010).

Simultaneous Use of a Long Cane and a Support Cane

If a client needs to learn to simultaneously use a long cane to probe the environment and a support cane for balance or strength, staying in-step and in-rhythm can be difficult. Being in-step with the cane implies that the student is moving the appropriate foot in time with the cane moving in the correct direction. Being in-rhythm refers to the cane and the foot contacting the

FIGURE 4.3

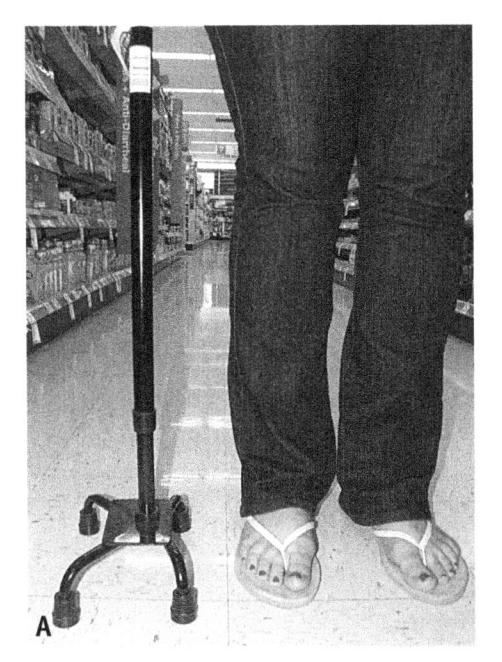

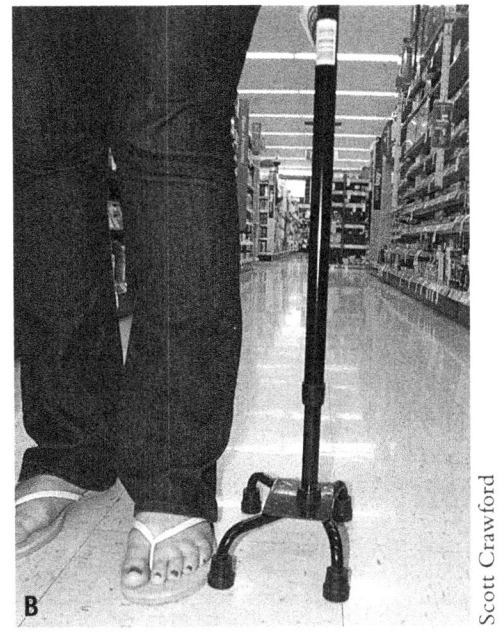

The feet of quad canes are set off-center from the shaft of the cane. When held correctly (**A**), the base of the cane does not interfere with travel. When held incorrectly (**B**), the feet of the cane become a tripping hazard.

ground or reaching the end of the arc at the same time. Determine first whether the support cane is to be used on the weaker or stronger side. For some clients, it will be helpful to first master staying in-step and in-rhythm with just the support cane. This can be done with either the two-point touch technique or the constant-contact technique. Human or voice guidance can be used until the client is ready to add the long cane.

If the support cane is used on the older adult's stronger side (and opposite the weaker side), the support cane should move forward with the leg on the opposite side of the body. Simultaneously, the long cane should swing toward the support cane (see Figure 4.4A). When the other leg moves forward, past the support cane, the long cane swings to the opposite side from the support cane (see Figure 4.4B). It helps clients to describe the movement as "canes together, canes apart."

If the support cane is on the older adult's weaker side, the support cane and the near leg (the weaker leg) should move at the same time. The long white cane moves to the opposite (stronger) side. As the support cane moves forward,

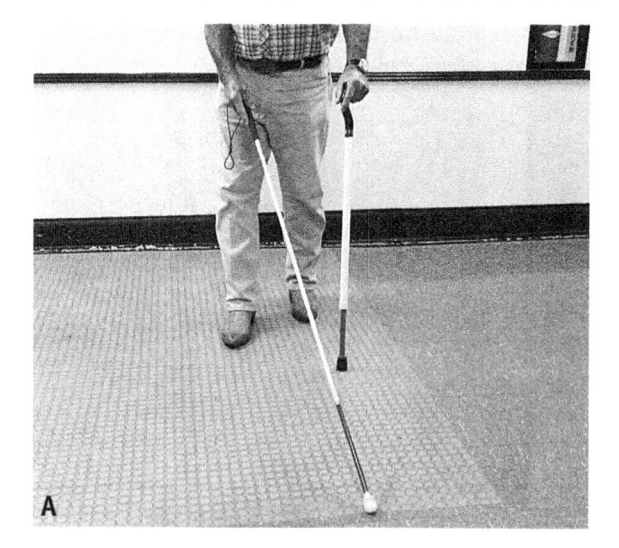

FIGURE **4.4**
"Canes together, canes apart." As the support cane moves forward in the opposite hand from the foot moving forward, the long cane moves toward the support cane (**A**). As the next step is taken and the client's body moves past the support cane, the long cane is swung away from the support cane (**B**).

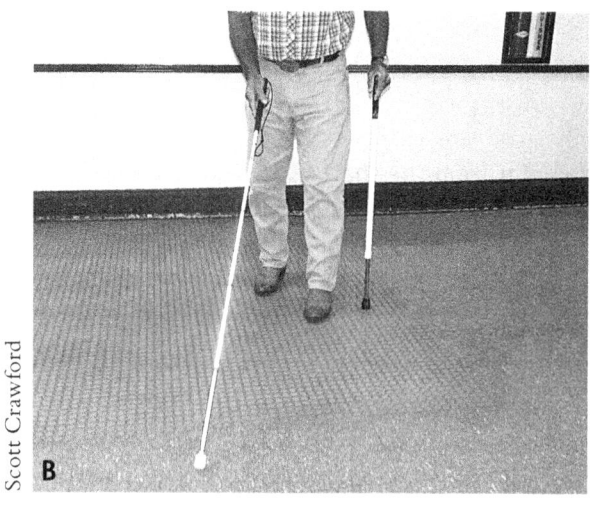

the long cane moves to the opposite side of the body (see Figure 4.5A). As the torso passes the support cane, the long cane moves to the same side as the support cane (see Figure 4.5B) (Rosen & Crawford, 2010). One way to describe the movement is "like windshield wipers." In this scenario, the two canes are never in the same place at the same time.

Using a Support Cane as a Probe

Some slow-moving older adults with short strides who can walk on flat surfaces without support can use support canes to probe the path in front of them.

FIGURE 4.5

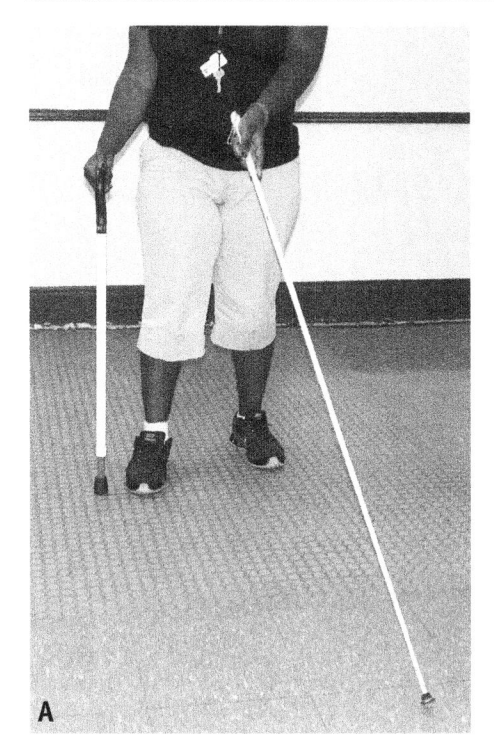

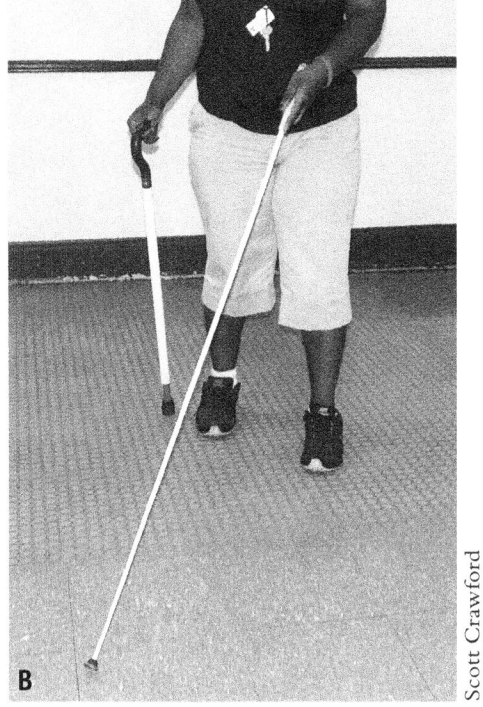

As the support cane moves forward on the same side as the foot moving forward, the long cane moves to the opposite side of the body (**A**). As the other foot moves forward, past the support cane, the long cane moves to the same side of the body as the support cane (**B**). The motion is similar to the movement of a car's windshield wipers.

Using the support cane as a probe can be effective for people who are able to stand and walk on smooth surfaces without support, but who may lose their balance when they walk on sloped surfaces, or who have a tendency to topple forward when stopping their stride. In these cases, the support cane is extended to the maximum length and the client uses the two-point touch technique (see Figure 4.6). Despite the short length of support canes, when the tip is extended in front of the trailing foot, it may still be a full stride ahead of the next foot placement. In some cases, the tip is more than one stride length ahead. If the older adult's foot lands beyond where the support cane tip touches, a different source of support may be needed. Alternatively, the older adult may be able to step forward with the support cane at the side of the

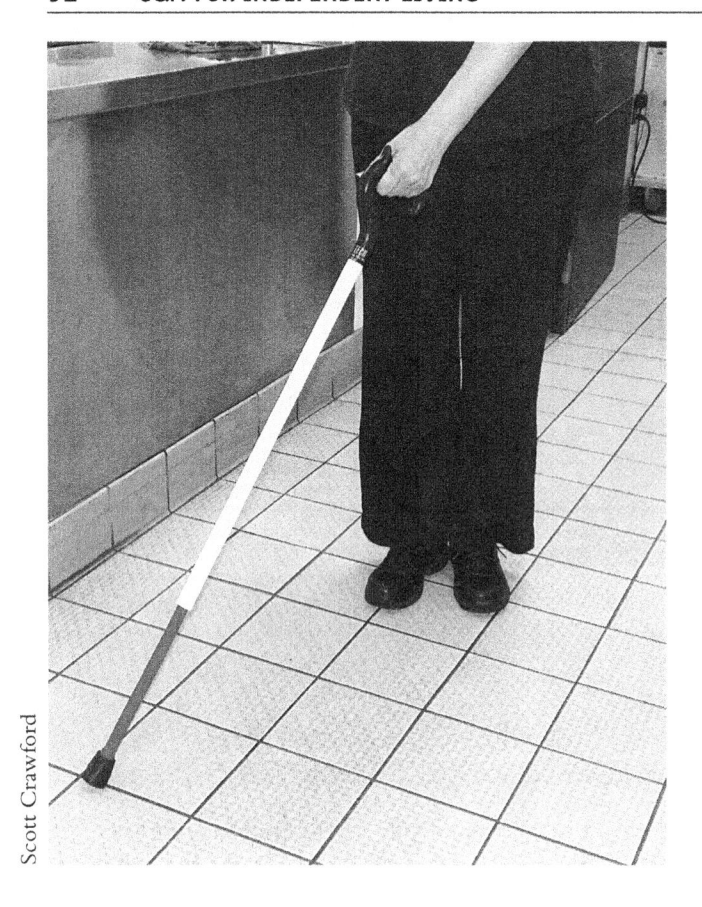

FIGURE **4.6**

Using a longer than standard support cane as a probe.

body, come to a complete stop, clear the path with the support cane, return the support cane to the side, and then take the next step forward (Crawford & Crawford, in press; Rosen & Crawford, 2010).

Using Two Support Canes

An older client who needs additional support may use a support cane in each hand (see Figure 4.7). The techniques are the same as those described for using a support cane and a long cane. The same support cane can be used to probe ahead each time, or the older adult can alternate canes. If only one of the canes is used to probe, it can be longer than the cane used for support. If alternating canes are used as the probe, both canes should be measured to provide maximum support for the older adult. When alternating canes, the cane moving forward also moves across the body to touch in front of the central line of the body (Figure 4.7A) and is then quickly moved to the side to be in

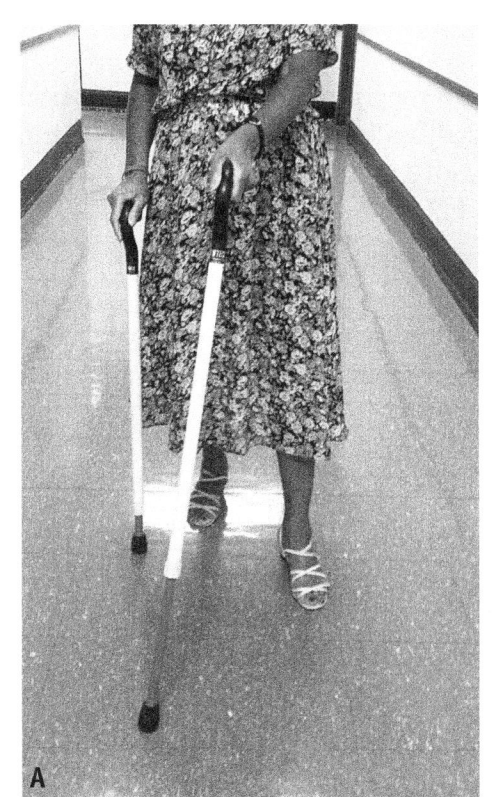

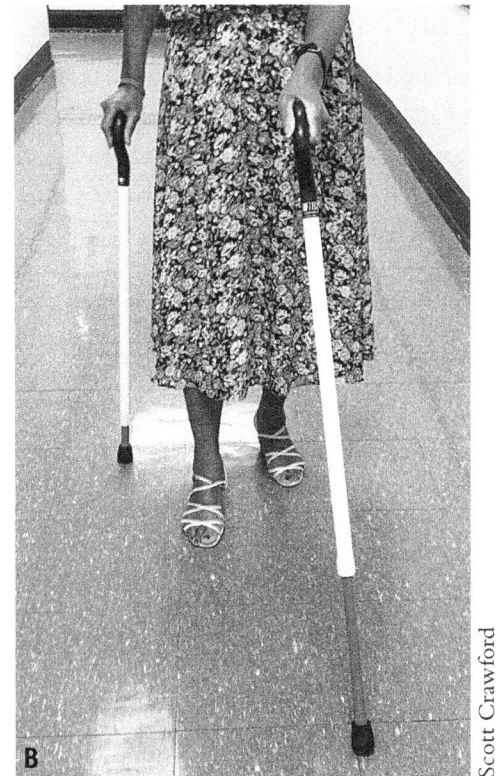

FIGURE **4.7**

When using two support canes, one can be used at the side of the body while the other is used in the two-point touch technique. Cane movement will follow the same patterns as if using a support cane and a long cane. When a support cane is used as a probe, it may not reach all the way across the body.

place for support as the older adult moves forward (Figure 4.7B). The second cane then repeats the movement from the other side. For most people in this scenario, neither support cane will reach all the way across the body. It is important that they at least reach to the center line of the user's body. Reaching too far across the body will reduce the forward reach of the cane and limit the older adult's reaction time. If the older adult's stride length puts his or her foot placement beyond where the cane tip touches, an alternative method for clearing the path may need to be found (Crawford & Crawford, in press; Rosen & Crawford, 2010).

Crutches

Standard crutches have handles, underarm supports, and one or two vertical shafts. Both the overall height of the crutch and the position of the hand grip can be adjusted. Forearm crutches do not have underarm supports. Instead, the hands grasp a handle that is attached to a long vertical shaft with plastic cuffs keep the forearms in place at the end of the crutch. (Rosen & Crawford, 2010).

The techniques used with crutches vary depending on the number of crutches used (one or two) and the degree to which the client can use his or

---

SIDEBAR 4.1

Walking with Crutches: Gait Patterns

Following are short summaries of the most common gait patterns for users of crutches.

SWING-TO GAIT

Weight is borne on better leg (or both if possible). Both crutches move forward at the same time. The body leans forward while the torso swings to a position even with the crutches.

SWING-THROUGH GAIT

Recommended sequence: Both crutches advance forward, then both legs are lifted off the ground and swung forward to land beyond the crutches.

TWO-POINT ALTERNATE CRUTCH GAIT

Right crutch and left foot move forward together, then left crutch and right foot move forward together.

Both crutches and the weaker leg move forward together, then the stronger leg moves forward.

FOUR-POINT ALTERNATE CRUTCH GAIT

Crutches and legs move individually and alternate in the following sequence:

1. Right crutch
2. Left foot
3. Left crutch
4. Right Foot

her own legs for support (see Sidebar 4.1 for common gait patterns used with crutches). When using two crutches, the crutches may advance at the same time, or they may alternate, moving in time with the opposite leg. As with any orthopedic device, crutches can be used all of the time, some of the time, or intermittently. The O&M specialist should consult with occupational and physical therapists to ensure that a specific technique can safely be used and to determine the appropriate gait pattern for the older adult.

Using a Crutch as a Probe

One modification for using two crutches without a long cane is to clear the path with the tip of one of the crutches before moving forward. The path can be cleared by first establishing balance (Figure 4.8A), then moving one of the crutches forward (Figure 4.8B). The other crutch then moves forward and across the body to touch the ground in front of the opposite foot (Figure 4.8C), before swinging back across the body and landing even with the first crutch (Figure 4.8D). The older adult then swings his or her body forward. With this technique, the feet should not swing past the line cleared by the crutches (Figure 4.8E). Older adults may clear the path with the same crutch each time, or if their balance permits, alternate crutches. Alternatively, older adults may clear the path with both crutches before each forward step. In this case, the first crutch moves straight forward. The second crutch then swings across the body and back to a forward position at the side of the path. The first crutch then swings across the body and then back to its forward position. The body is then swung forward, not passing the line cleared by the crutches.

Guiding Techniques with Crutches

Older adults with crutches can be guided by voice or by using the reverse human guide technique, in which the guide holds the traveler's elbow. The guide applies gentle pressure to the traveler's arm to steer the traveler in the desired direction. If using the reverse human guide technique, the guide's touch needs to be very light to ensure that the traveler has as much freedom of movement as possible. The guide may apply light pressure to the traveler's arm, but should not physically move the traveler's arm in any direction. All movement should be initiated by the older adult. Tightening the grasp and pulling back lightly can indicate the need to stop.

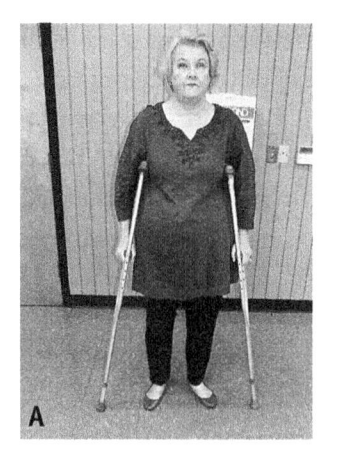

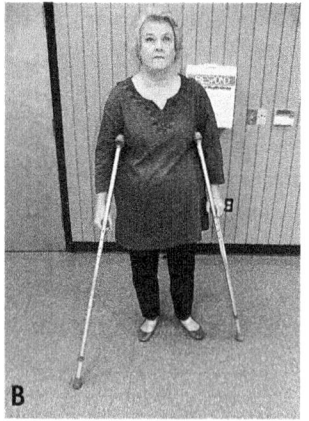

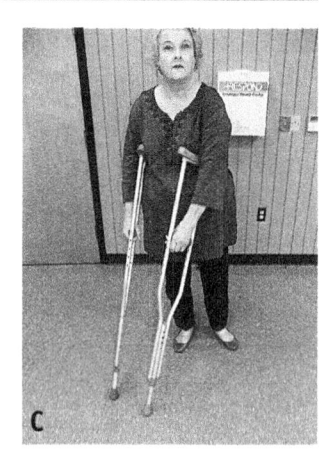

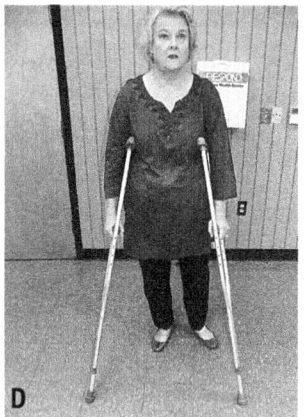

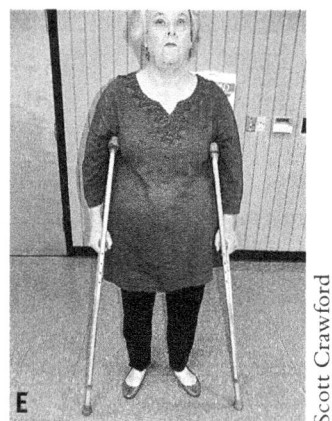

FIGURE **4.8**
Using two crutches as pathway probes can be an arduous process.

Using Crutches with a Long White Cane

If an older adult has large enough hands and a strong enough grip, it may be possible for him or her to use crutches and a long white cane at the same time. To do so, the client uses one hand to grasp both the cane and the handle of one of his or her crutches. The client may grasp the cane with the index and middle fingers of one hand and grasp the crutch handle with the thumb, ring, and pinky fingers, keeping most of the weight on the palm of the hand (see Figure 4.9). The cane is then swung back and forth, using a twist of the radius and ulna (the same motion as turning a door knob) (see Figure 4.10).

A slower method is for the older adult to come to a complete stop, let go of the crutch with the hand holding the cane, clear the path with the cane,

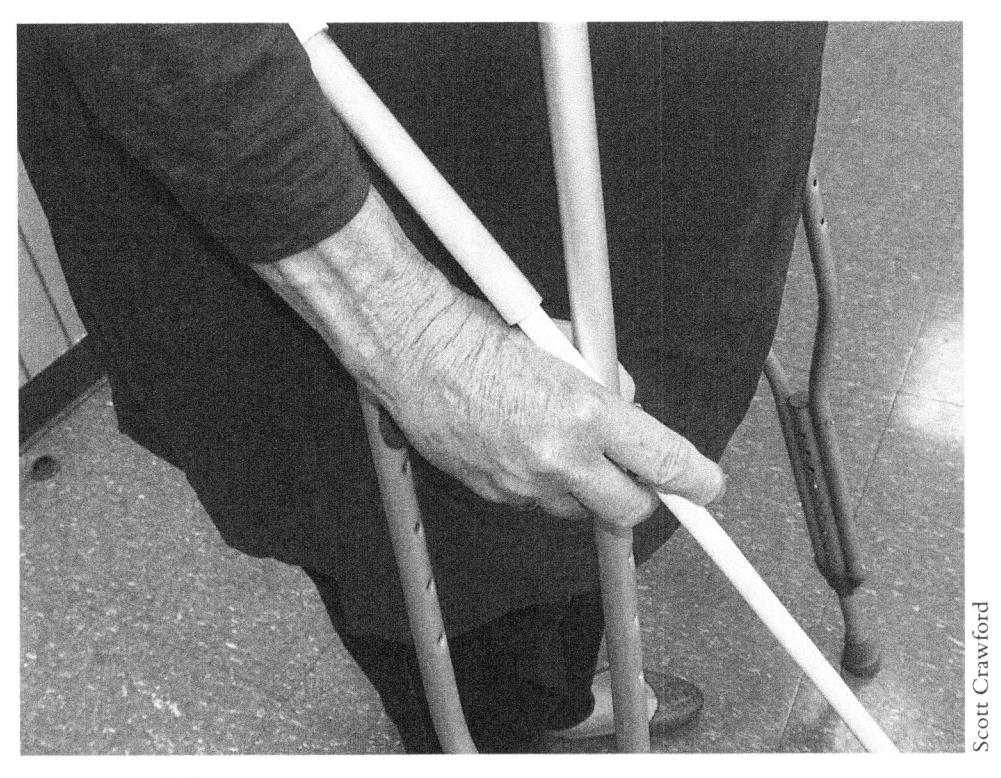

FIGURE 4.9
The client can hold the cane with the index and middle finger (as shown here) or use all four fingers to hold the handle of the cane next to the handle of the crutch. Holding the cane at the very end of the handle allows for a wider sweep with the cane.

re-grasp the crutch handle, and finally, move forward. This is a tedious method of travel but may provide the best combination of support and path clearance.

Walkers

As with support canes, determining the medical need to use a walker falls outside of the scope of O&M specialists. If an older adult has been instructed by a physical therapist, occupational therapist, or physician to use a walker, O&M specialists need to support that recommendation.

Standard Walkers

Standard walkers, also known as medical walkers or hospital walkers, provide solid support for the older adult while also providing a bumper that can

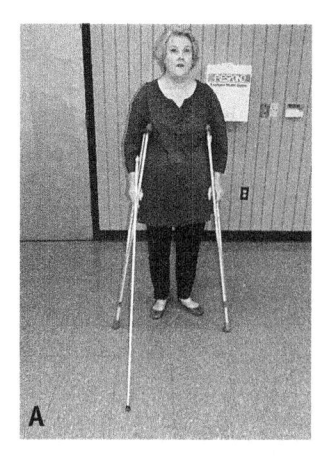

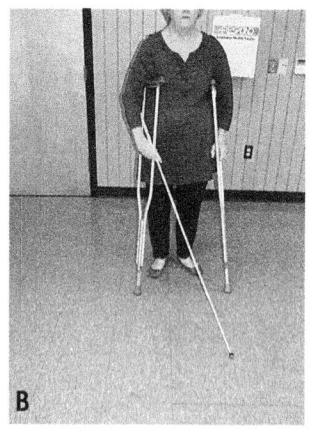

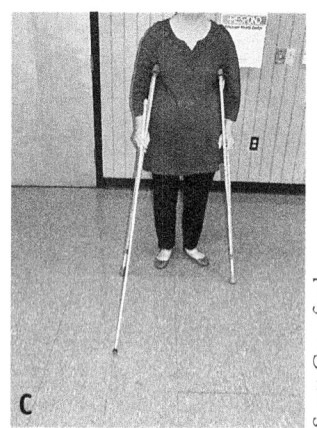

FIGURE 4.10
People who have the manual dexterity and grip strength can hold the cane in one of their hands while also holding onto their crutches. A radial-ulnar twist will swing the cane across the body.

be utilized to probe the environment. Standard walkers usually have four legs attached to a metal frame that wraps around the front of the traveler, with an opening at the traveler's back. For maximum support, all legs of the walker should be capped with rubber feet to keep the walker from slipping. If a traveler has trouble lifting the walker, wheels may be added to the front legs so that lifting just the back two legs allows the walker to roll forward. Another common modification is to add tennis balls to the back two legs, which allows the walker to slide forward without lifting.

Reverse Walkers

Reverse walkers are similar to standard walkers except they wrap around the back of the traveler and have the opening in front (see Figure 4.11). These types of walkers provide the highest degree of support and are more often used with children than adults. Reverse walkers are deeper than standard front walkers, with the sides extending forward beyond the traveler, in a configuration resembling three sides of a square. This design keeps the traveler between the sides of the walker, even when moving. When using standard walkers and rollators (discussed in the next section), people often allow the walker to proceed too far in front of them, severely reducing the amount of support the walker provides. The design of the reverse walker prevents a similar situation from occurring. Reverse walkers can have zero, two, or four

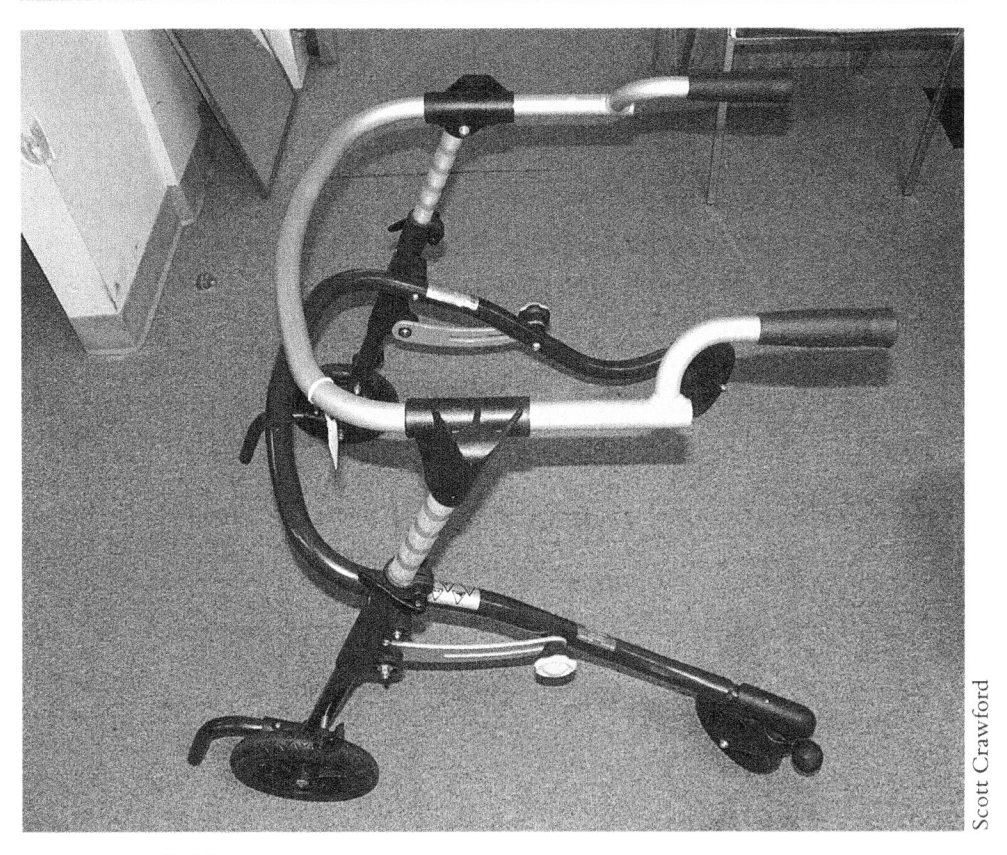

FIGURE **4.11**
Reverse walkers wrap behind the traveler and can be used by adults who need extra support when traveling.

wheels, and the wheels can be set to swivel or stay static. The wheels may also be designed to roll in only one direction, which prevents the walker from rolling backwards unintentionally.

Rollators

Rollators, or four-wheeled walkers, provide the least amount of support for the older adult. In a typical setup, two wheels of a rollator move forward and backward only, and two wheels are caster wheels that can move in any direction. The location (front or back) of the casters affects both the level of support and how the older adult must move when making turns. Clients should try walkers with both locations for the casters to determine which provides the best balance of support and maneuverability. Many rollators have built-in seats that travelers can use for resting.

Knee Walkers

Knee walkers resemble a child's scooter. These devices can be very helpful to people with problems in their lower legs. To use a knee walker, the traveler kneels on the cushion of the walker with his or her weaker leg, holds the handlebars, and moves the walker forward or back by pushing with the healthier leg (see Figure 4.12). The device is steered by the handlebars.

If a long white cane is needed, the older adult can hold the handlebars with one hand and use the other hand to hold the cane. The cane can be held in a centered position above the handlebars, or the stronger hand can hold the cane below the handlebars, sweeping the cane across the front of the knee walker.

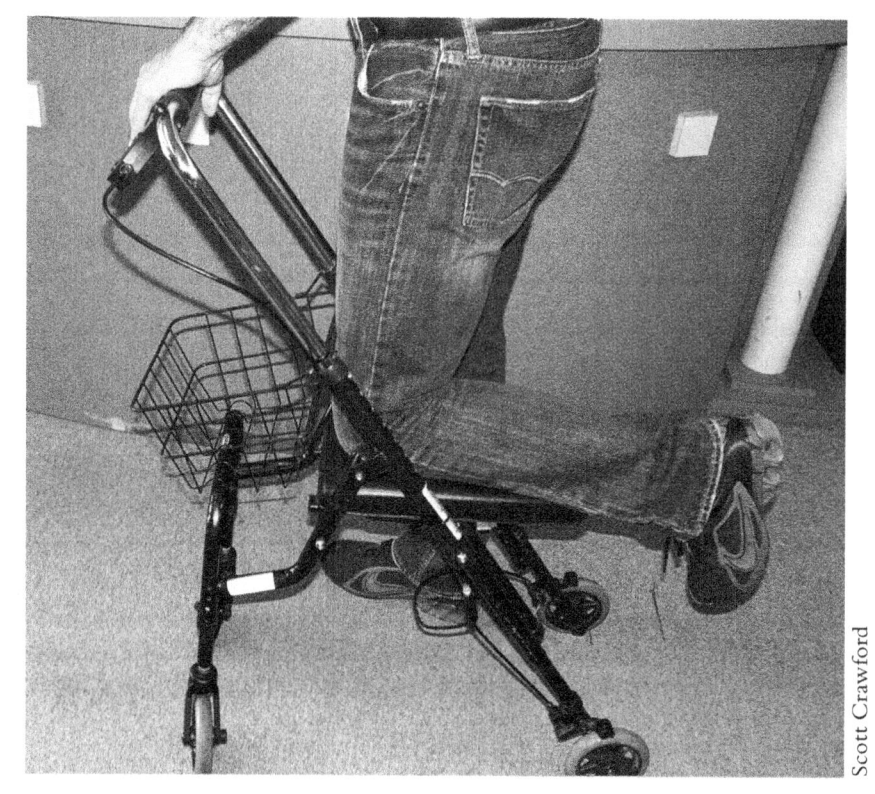

FIGURE **4.12**
Knee walkers allow the traveler to kneel on a base, taking all the body weight off of the lower leg, ankle, or foot.

Guiding Techniques for Walkers

If the older adult is stable enough to hold the walker with just one hand, the human guide techniques for older adults with walkers can be similar to those used with travelers in wheelchairs (discussed later in this chapter). The best grasp for guiding when using a walker with one hand is for the traveler to put a hand on top of the guide's forearm. For turns toward the older adult, the guide can point the forearm across the older adult's body to indicate the turn. For walking single file or navigating doorways, the guide may have to turn around, face the older adult, and back through the opening or narrow passage. If the older adult needs the added support of keeping both hands on the handlebars, using the reverse human guide technique can be effective (see Figure 4.13).

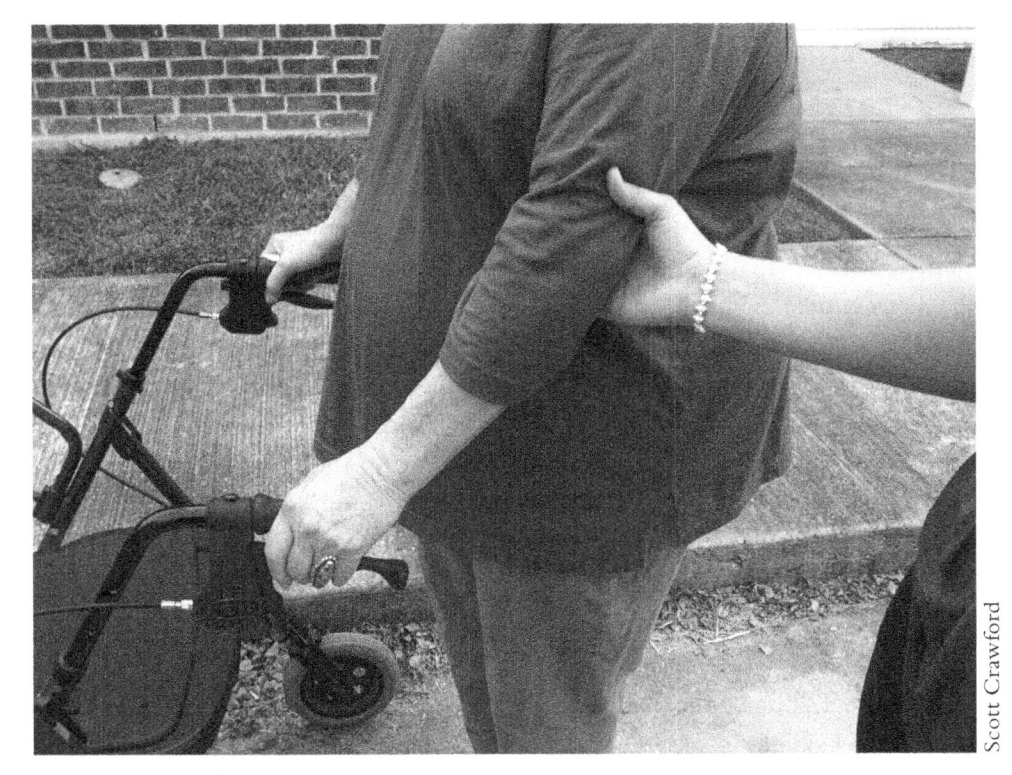

FIGURE **4.13**
The reverse human guide technique allows the traveler to keep both hands free to utilize mobility devices. The guide lightly grasps the traveler's elbow and only uses very gentle pressure.

Another alternative is for the guide to grasp one of the front corners of the walker and steer the walker. Caution must be taken to not move the walker faster than the older adult can move. If the older adult controls the forward momentum of the walker, the guide can push or pull the front of the walker to adjust the line of travel and stop forward momentum if there is an obstacle in front of the older adult.

Navigating Curbs with Walkers

Locating the Curb or Drop-Off. The first step in navigating curbs when using a walker is locating the curb or drop-off. People who are able to see drop-offs and obstacles can walk and move the walker at the same time. If the older adult needs support from a walker and does not have depth perception to see the drop-off, he or she either needs to use a cane (discussed in the next section) or the "Walker Waltz" technique (named for its three steps), described in Sidebar 4.2. In the "Walker Waltz," either the traveler's feet can move, or the walker can move, but never both at the same time.

Negotiating Drop-Offs. There are several ways to approach a drop-off. Once a drop-off is located, the traveler can negotiate the change in level by moving forward, moving backward, or moving sideways. The method will depend on the client's ability to lean forward slightly and lift the walker.

For *forward navigation,* the client will locate the edge of the drop-off, align the direction of travel to be perpendicular to the edge, and move the walker up to, but not over, the edge. To do so, the client may have to lean the walker over the edge and then pull it back until all of the feet on the walker are stable. The client then steps as close to the edge of the drop-off as the walker will allow (ideally, right at the edge). Next, the client lifts the walker, swings the back legs forward until they clear the edge, leans forward, and lowers the walker to the ground. A degree of strength is required to lean forward enough for the walker to reach the bottom without the individual falling forward, and some older adults will need assistance with lowering the walker off the drop-off. The client then steps down with the weaker side, which allows the stronger side to lower the client's body weight to the ground. Some people have an easier time with this movement if they turn their body slightly toward the stronger side. When doing so, the body should turn less than 90 degrees, or else after the first step there won't be enough room between the first foot and the curb to accommodate the second foot. The walker should always remain perpendicular to the edge, regardless of body position.

SIDEBAR 4.2

The Walker Waltz Technique for Traveling with a Walker

When older adults who use walkers are unable to visually maintain their safety or to use a cane to reliably probe the environment, they risk tipping the walker at cracks or drop-offs. To utilize the walker as a probe for the environment, older adults should adopt a gait pattern referred to as the "Walker Waltz." As always, it is important for the O&M specialist to consult with a client's physical therapist to ensure the highest degree of safety before teaching a new technique.

1. With feet planted at shoulder width, the client moves the walker forward, stops the walker, and then gives the walker a little wiggle to make sure all four feet are on the ground. (If a drop-off is approached at an angle, it may be difficult to detect if one of the feet of the walker is dangling off the edge. Wiggling the walker is the best way to test for this.)

2. If the walker is stable, the older adult then steps forward with one leg. (If the client has a weaker side, he or she should step forward first with that side, unless a physical or occupational therapist has directed otherwise, so that the individual's torso is further into the walker and has more support when the weight is on the weaker side.)

3. The older adult then steps forward with the other leg. It can be a "step, together" type step (as in a two-step dance). Some people may be able to pass the first leg with the second, while others may need to keep the second leg just behind the first leg. Once the second leg has moved, the older adult will need a moment to reestablish balance before moving the walker again.

The older adult then repeats steps 1, 2, and 3 (hence the waltz reference) until the drop-off, curb, or other obstacle is located. The traveler should advance the walker slowly so that he or she has time to react to tilts and level changes. Some older adults will need to use this technique anytime they are in unfamiliar environments or in familiar environments with known obstacles and hazards.

Sideways navigation of curbs and single drop-offs can be an option for people who cannot bend over to lower the walker to ground level. The edge is detected as in the forward navigation technique. The traveler then turns the walker toward the stronger side. The walker should be turned 90 degrees or, ideally, 120 to 135 degrees. The traveler then sidesteps to the edge of the drop-off, bringing the feet as close together as possible before stepping down with the weaker side leg (see Figure 4.14). The foot stepping down either needs to be angled so that the second foot has somewhere to land, or the traveler needs to step out far enough that there is room for the second foot between the first foot and the curb. Usually, people who need to step down sideways do not have the strength or balance to step far enough away from the curb. Angling the first foot so the toe is pointed at the curb and the heel away from the curb will allow the torso to remain facing the walker. Once both feet are on the ground there are two choices: (1) the traveler can lift the walker and turn away from the curb to bring it to ground level; or (2) the traveler can turn to face

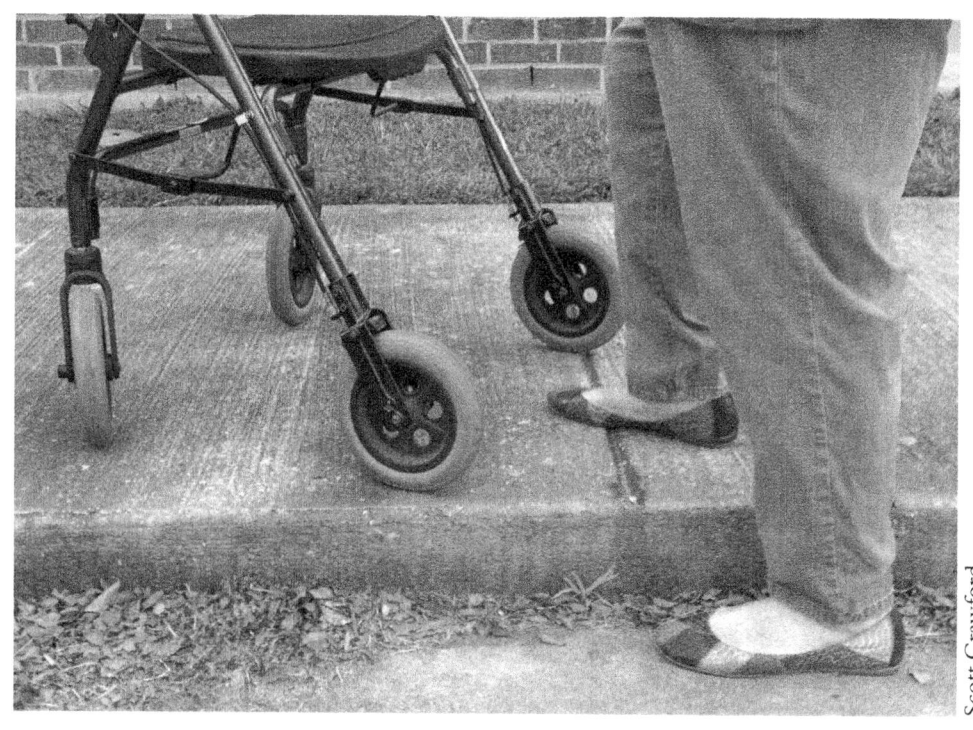

FIGURE **4.14**
Clients who do not have the physical ability to step forward off of a curb with a walker may be able to step off sideways.

the curb, turn the walker to face away from the drop-off (aligning the back of the walker with the edge), back up slightly (just enough to make room for the walker), lower the back legs of the walker to ground level, take another step back to make room for the walker (if necessary), and finally, pull the walker over the edge to lower the front legs to the ground.

The method of descending curbs that provides the most support is *going down backward*. With this technique, the traveler does not have to let go of the walker or bend over while facing forward. The traveler locates the drop-off as described earlier, gets as close to the edge as possible, then turns his or her body and the walker 180 degrees. Now, the traveler's back is to the drop-off. The traveler then slides the weaker foot backward to feel for the edge, so that the stronger leg can hold the traveler's weight during this process. If the traveler is not yet at the edge, he or she plants the foot to step backward and probes again. Once the edge has been located, the traveler pulls the walker back until its back legs are at the edge of the drop-off. The traveler then steps down with the weaker leg first, which allows the stronger leg to lower his or her weight to the ground (see Figure 4.15). Once both feet are on the ground, the steps are the same as described for the sideways technique.

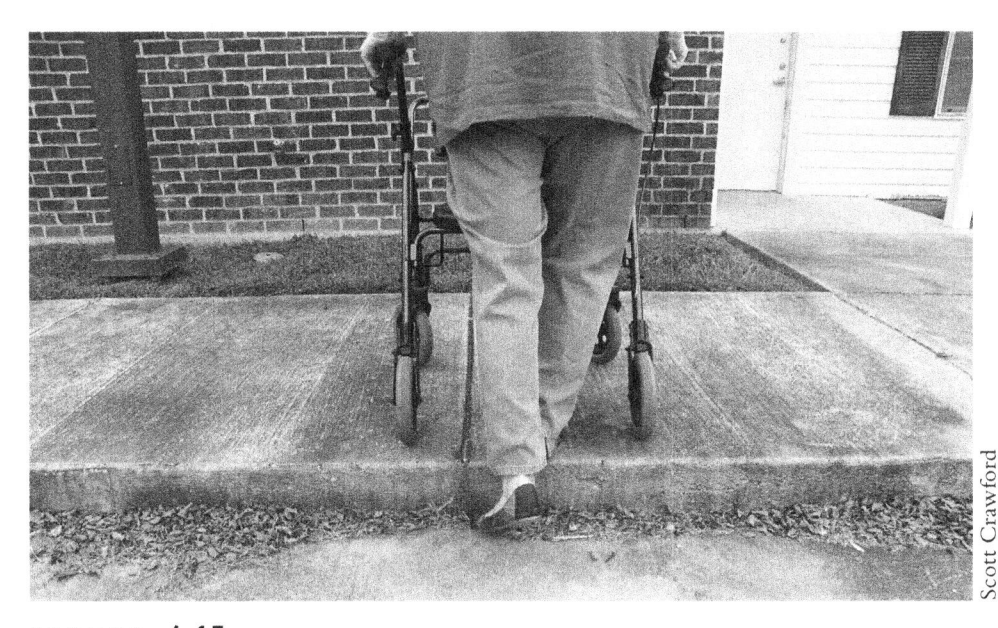

FIGURE **4.15**
Some clients may have to step off of curbs backward when using a walker. The drop-off should be located while facing forward, then the client should turn around to step off.

Stepping up with a Walker. Older adults who use walkers should always step up while facing forward. The stronger side steps up first so the traveler does not have to lift his or her body weight with the weaker leg.

Using a Walker with a Long White Cane

People with some hand dexterity can hold a cane and the handle of a walker at the same time (see Figure 4.16A). Usually, the cane is held in the fingertips and the palm is resting on the handle of the walker. The pencil grasp (Figure 4.16B) allows the student to put weight on the palm and use the thumb, index, and middle fingers to hold the cane. The ring and pinky fingers grasp the walker handle.

Some people can swing the cane and walk at the same time. Others may have to alternate walking two or three steps with standing still to clear the path with the cane. The number of steps taken should not exceed the distance that the cane has cleared. To determine the number of steps that should be used, have the client face a wall or line on the floor. Position the client far enough back that the cane swipe just barely hits the wall or line on the floor. Then have the client walk forward and count the number of steps it takes to

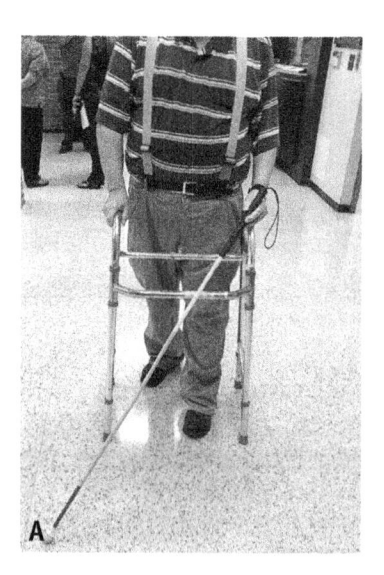

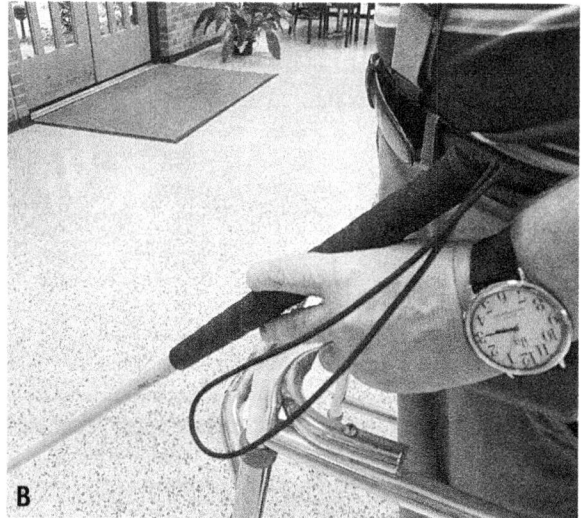

FIGURE **4.16**
Clients can use a walker with long cane (**A**) by holding the long cane in a pencil grasp (**B**).

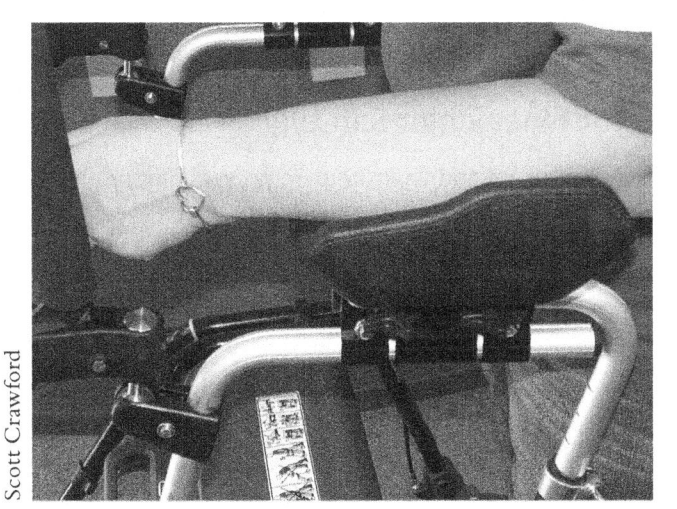

FIGURE **4.17**

Forearm rests can replace one or both handles on a walker, allowing a free hand to swing a long white cane.

Scott Crawford

reach the wall or cross the line. Subtract one step to arrive at the number of steps the client can safely take between swings with the cane.

On most walkers, one of the handles can be replaced by a forearm rest (see Figure 4.17) on which the older adult can lean, leaving one of the hands free to hold a long cane. Using this position requires the approval of the client's physical therapist or occupational therapist. Using this position without consulting these related service professionals could leave the client at risk for injury and the O&M specialist open to unnecessary liability.

Wheelchairs

It has been reported that as many as 1 in 10 people with visual impairments will have to use a wheelchair at some point in their lives (Ivanchenko, Coughlan, Gerrey, & Shen, 2008). An older adult may need a wheelchair intermittently or consistently, for brief periods of time, or for extended periods of time. For example, an athlete who is blind may sustain an injury that requires the use of a wheelchair for a period of days, weeks, or months; once healed, he or she may never need a wheelchair again. An individual with diabetes or multiple sclerosis may have repeated periodic incidents during which a wheelchair is required for short periods of time (Crawford & Crawford, in press). O&M specialists will want all clients who use wheelchairs, regardless of the type of chair, to be familiar with the rules for wheelchair safety (see Sidebar 4.3).

SIDEBAR 4.3

Rules for Wheelchair Safety

The following rules for wheelchair users and their helpers prevent injury and facilitate orientation.

RULE #1: BRAKES.

Any time the wheelchair user gets in or out of the chair, the brakes should be on. Powered devices should be turned off. When stationary, it is still better to engage the brakes on an uneven surface. The chair could roll, causing the student to lose his or her orientation.

For example: A buxom elderly wheelchair user leaned forward as she was trying to get out of her powered chair. In the process, the joystick was pushed forward, causing the chair to lurch forward.

Another wheelchair user, while reaching for the arm rest to help her sit down, instead grabbed the joystick, causing the chair to move backwards, leaving her sitting on the footrest.

RULE #2: ASK BEFORE YOU PUSH.

If a helper pushes the wheelchair without warning, he or she may accidentally cause injury to the user.

For example: A wheelchair user was struggling with a steep curb ramp. Another pedestrian noticed his struggle, stepped behind the wheelchair, and gave it a big push. Unfortunately, the wheelchair user's pinky was caught between the wheel and the wheel rail and the user was injured.

RULE #3: DON'T LET GO!

Visually impaired wheelchair users will have a harder time maintaining their orientation if they release the wheel rails while moving. They should come to a complete stop, then let go of the wheel rails.

When pushing wheelchairs, helpers should not let go of the chair's handles before telling the wheelchair user.

For example: As a staff member pushed a visually impaired wheelchair user out of the building for a fire drill, she noticed another patient struggling with the door. The staff member left the wheelchair user sitting on the building ramp as she turned to help the other patient. Gravity propelled the wheelchair user down the ramp and into the person standing in front of the user.

RULE #4: IF YOUR WHEELS ARE MOVING, YOUR CANE SHOULD BE MOVING.

For wheelchair users that also use a long white cane, it is important to use the cane to clear the path any time the chair is moving.

RULE #5: NEVER CENTER THE CANE.

Wheelchairs, whether powered or not, cannot stop as quickly as a person that is walking. If the cane becomes stuck while centered, the handle can be driven into the user's torso, or up into the face.

RULE #6: DON'T STEP OVER THE FOOTREST.

Any time a person steps in our out of the chair, the footrest should be moved out of the way to ease the transition. Trying to step over the footrests while getting in or out of the chair can cause a person to lose his or her balance and fall.

RULE #7: CASTERS FORWARD BEFORE STANDING UP.

By moving the casters forward before standing up, additional support is provided to the front of the chair, reducing the probability of the chair tipping forward as the user stands.

RULE #8: NEVER DRINK AND DRIVE.

In addition to illegal drugs and alcohol, prescribed medications can have an adverse effect on the wheelchair user's ability to safely and efficiently operate the wheelchair. Fatigue, low blood sugar, and other health problems can also be an issue.

RULE #9: IF YOU'RE NOT SURE, DON'T GO.

Whether crossing a street, navigating around an obstacle, or just going out the door, if the older adult is not 100% certain of being safe, he or she should not go.

RULE #10: NO PASSENGERS.

Wheelchair users sometimes decide to provide rides to friends or family members. While fun, riders make it more difficult to independently maintain orientation and safety. Riders can be thrown from the chair, become wedged between the chair and an obstacle, or damage the chair.

Types of Wheelchairs

There are many different types of wheelchairs. Table 4.1 summarizes the advantages and disadvantages of the types most commonly used by older adults who are visually impaired.

Hospital and Transport Wheelchairs. Hospital and transport wheelchairs must be pushed by an attendant because none of the wheels are large enough to be reached by the person being transported. Some are designed like adult-sized strollers.

Sports Wheelchairs. Some wheelchairs are modified for athletic competition. The tops of the large wheels are tilted in towards the chair, creating a wider base (/-\) that provides additional support during turns and reduces the chances of tipping. The footrests and front wheels are shortened and sometimes rounded so that the chair needs less space for turning. The footrests may be positioned so that the user's knees are bent more than 90 degrees, partially tucking the feet under the seat, which can greatly reduce the amount of space needed for turning.

Powered Wheelchairs. Wheelchairs and other mobility devices that run on batteries are now referred to as powered mobility devices (the term "electric chair" is no longer accepted in the professional world). Most powered mobility devices are operated by a joystick—a lever that can move around in all directions to control the movement of the wheels—but they can also be operated by a wide variety of alternative methods. People who cannot utilize joysticks to operate a device can use head arrays, chin controls, and suck-and-blow systems, among other options. There is even an iPhone application that can be used to operate a powered wheelchair (Crawford & Crawford, in press).

Scooters. Electric scooters are the least expensive form of a powered mobility device, with some models costing less than $1,000. Scooters have a tiller (handlebars) in the front, a platform for the feet behind the tiller, and a seat that is usually situated over the drive motor toward the rear of the device. Most scooters can be driven with either hand. Most cane users find it easier to drive with the right hand and swing the cane with the left. If the user can reach under the handlebars with the cane hand, the cane can swing completely across the path. O&M specialists will want to teach older clients to drive both forward and backward with either hand.

TABLE 4.1 Advantages and Disadvantages of Wheelchairs, Power Chairs, and Scooters

Characteristic	Manual Wheelchair	Power Wheelchair	Scooter
Maneuverability	Turns easily in tight spaces	Turns easily in tight spaces	Larger turning radius
Steering	Difficult to maintain line of travel without vision	Difficult to maintain line of travel; can have overly sensitive controls	Easy to maintain straight line of travel
Cost	Can be the cheapest option, but personalization may significantly increase cost	Frequently more expensive than other options	Less expensive than power wheelchairs
Stamina	Requires more physical effort and can be physically taxing; exercise can enhance consumer health	Requires less physical strength to operate	Requires less physical strength to operate
Portability	Easily placed in vehicles and easily carried up and down stairs	Special transportation required	Can be disassembled and placed in standard vehicles
Personalization	Seating and positioning systems can be added if needed	Seating and positioning systems can be added if needed	Cannot add supports if user needs trunk support
Protection			Tiller (handlebars) and front structure creates a barrier between the user and obstacles
Procurement	Any doctor can prescribe	Any doctor can prescribe	Not recommended by many physical therapists; only certain types of doctors can recommend
Use with cane	Can be difficult to push the chair and utilize a long white cane at the same time	Can have one hand free for cane use	Can have one hand free for cane use

Many older adults with severely impaired vision prefer scooters. If the primary source of information is the cane, it is easier to recognize and maintain a straight line of travel with the scooter's tiller than with the joystick on powered wheelchairs. The tiller can also act as a barrier in front of the user. Scooters can be disassembled and put into the trunk of a car for transport, alleviating the need for lifts or ramped vehicles.

Propulsion of Manual Chairs. Manual chairs can be propelled using the hands or the feet. Without visual references to maintain orientation, it can be extremely difficult to propel the chair with the hands in a desired line of travel. If older clients have any use of their legs, keeping a foot on the ground can help keep the chair moving in straight line (see Figure 4.18). Using a foot to propel the chair can also leave a hand free to utilize a long cane.

For cane users with manual wheelchairs who cannot use their legs, there are several options to propel the chair including the following:

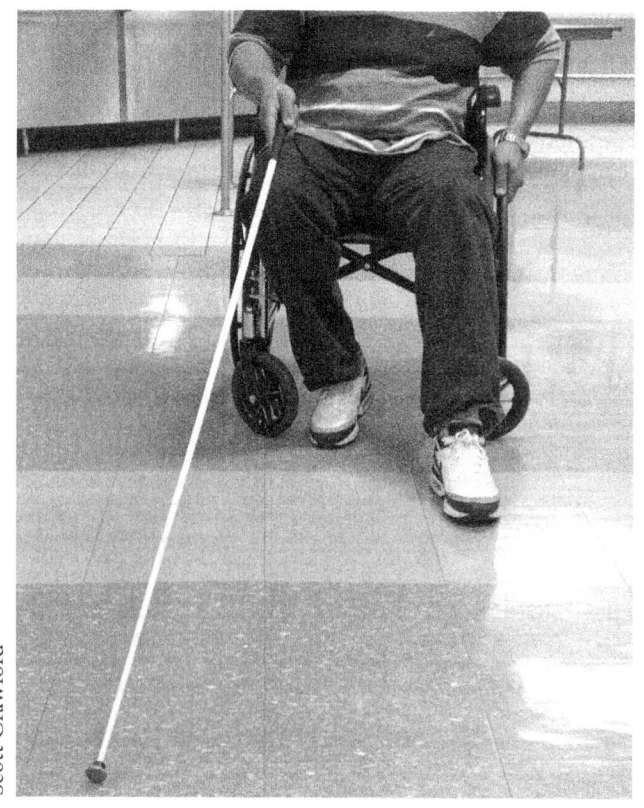

FIGURE **4.18**
Clients who can use their feet to assist with propelling the wheelchair will have an easier time maintaining a straight line of travel.

1. The user can grasp the cane and the wheel rail with one hand. After the wheel is pushed forward and released, the cane then clears the path before the rail is re-grasped.
2. The user can push one wheel forward, change the cane to the opposite hand, and then use the free hand to push the second wheel.
3. The user can keep the cane in one hand while the other hand alternates pushing each wheel. Often, the push that is made when reaching across the body is weaker than the push made on the same side. To help maintain a straight line of travel, older adults may push twice on the weaker side for each push on the stronger side.

Guiding Techniques for People in Wheelchairs

Guiding a client in a wheelchair is different than guiding a client who is ambulatory. While the obvious solution for guiding a person in a wheelchair seems to be to push the chair, in some cases that is not possible. For powered devices, pushing can be very difficult and should only be done when the device has broken down for one reason or another. As a general rule, a wheelchair should never be pushed by a helper unless permission has been granted by the wheelchair user and the individual has moved his or her hands away from the wheels. For guiding powered devices, either the older adult can hold the guide's forearm, as shown in Figure 4.19, or the guide can drive the chair by using the joystick or tiller while walking alongside the chair. When being guided, a client in a wheelchair should place his or her hand on top of the human guide's forearm instead of above the elbow (Figure 4.19A).

When the client holds the guide's forearm, additional distance is allowed between the guide and the front wheels of the chair. To make a turn toward the chair, the guide may need to point across the older adult's body with the grasped forearm. The guide can turn around to face the older adult and back out through narrow passages and doorways (Figure 4.19B). If the older adult does not react to the guide stopping, the guide can lift the hand of the held arm into a halt position (Figure 4.19C). The exaggerated motion will usually be dramatic enough for the client to recognize the signal.

If the guide is going to drive the chair, the speed controls should be turned down to a speed slow enough that the guide can push the control fully forward and still maintain a comfortable walking pace. For scooters, it is easiest if the guide drives from the right side of the scooter so that the throttle control lever is being pushed forward instead of having to be pulled back as it

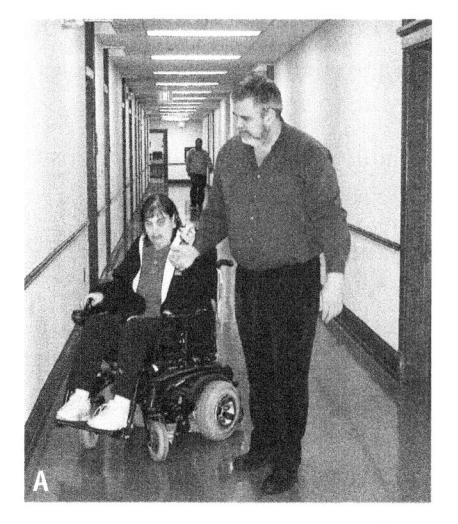

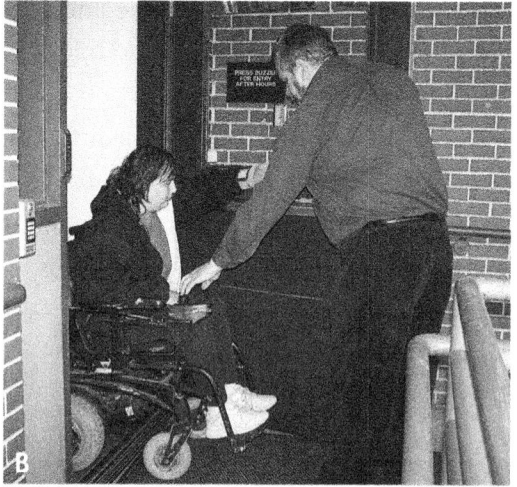

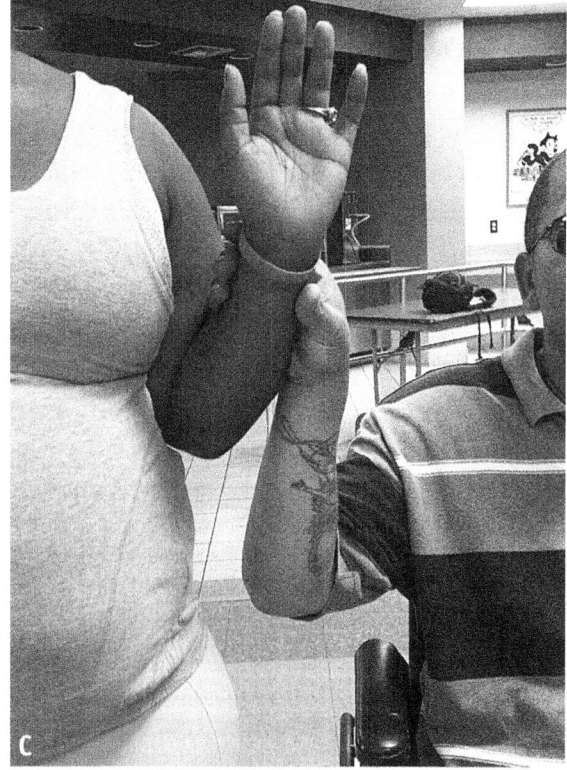

FIGURE **4.19**

Guiding a client in a wheelchair (**A**), backing through a narrow doorway (**B**), and raising an arm to signal "stop" (**C**).

would have to be if driving on the left. Again, for narrow passages and doorways, the guide can turn around to face the older adult and back through the opening. The older adult should be taught to reach out and assist with holding doors open until the chair has cleared the doorway.

Using a Wheelchair with a Long White Cane

Using the long cane with wheelchairs is different from using it while walking. The first major difference is that the cane should never be centered. Wheelchairs do not stop immediately, and if the cane should get stuck while the chair is moving, the wheelchair user could be injured by the cane. Instead, the hand holding the cane should be kept to the side so if the cane gets stuck and the chair continues moving, the top of the cane has a better chance of missing the wheelchair user's torso or face. Most older adults prefer to use the constant-contact technique rather than the two-point touch technique when in a wheelchair. Small cracks and drop-offs that may have little effect on ambulatory older adults may be more of a problem for wheelchair users.

Cane length is a major factor in how fast the older adult can operate the wheelchair. Wheelchair users need the longest cane they can effectively manage. Longer canes can feel extremely heavy, especially to people whose strength and stamina are limited by additional disabilities.

When the wheelchair user is backing up, the cane needs to be turned around to clear the path behind the wheelchair or scooter (see Figure 4.20). For older adults with low vision, mirrors can also be attached to the chair to show what is immediately behind it.

Navigating Tight Spaces and Turns

One of the major issues with training a wheelchair user with vision loss is navigating through turns and narrow passages. Before working with actual doorways or on sidewalks, it is recommended that the skills be introduced through practice in navigating in between two easily movable obstacles, such as chairs or lightweight trash cans (see Figure 4.21). That way, when errors are made, the obstacles will move instead of being damaged or causing damage to the wheelchair. With practice, many older adults can become familiar with landmarks on either the wheelchair or a body part that can be used to help indicate when to turn. For example, a wheelchair user may drive parallel to the wall until arriving in front of an open doorway. The user knows that when the joystick is even with the doorjamb on the far side of the opening, the chair is lined up to make a crisp 90-degree turn, after which the user will

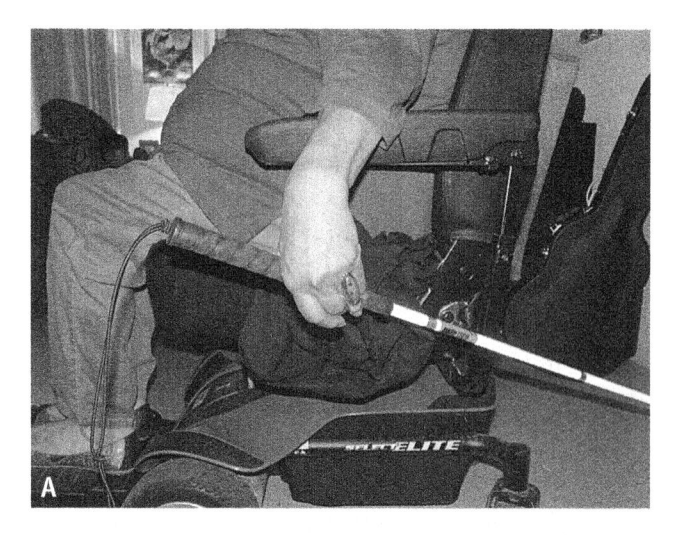

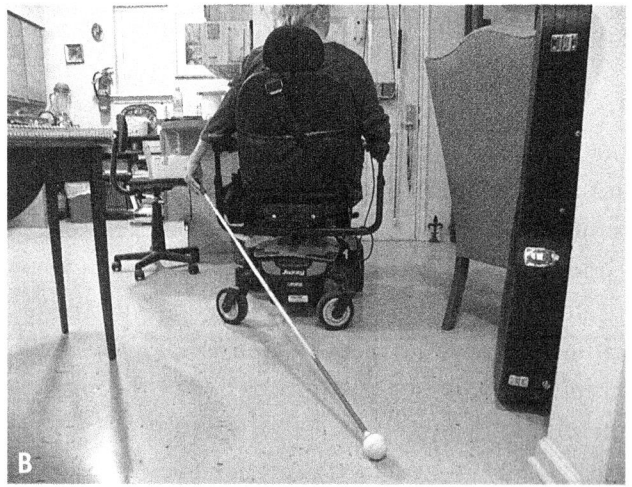

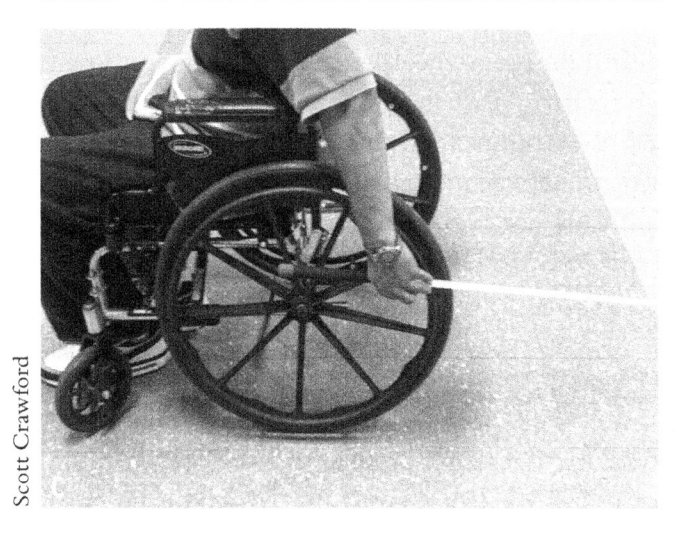

FIGURE **4.20**

Several views of using the long cane repositioned to clear the area behind a wheelchair before backing up.

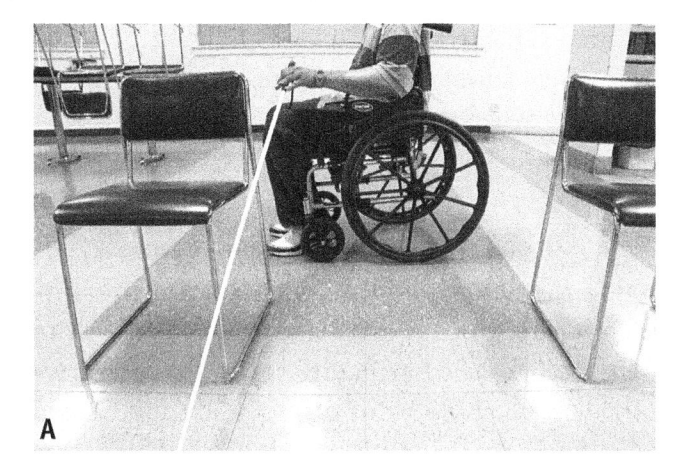

FIGURE **4.21**
Navigation skills can be introduced through practice in navigating in between movable obstacles such as chairs.

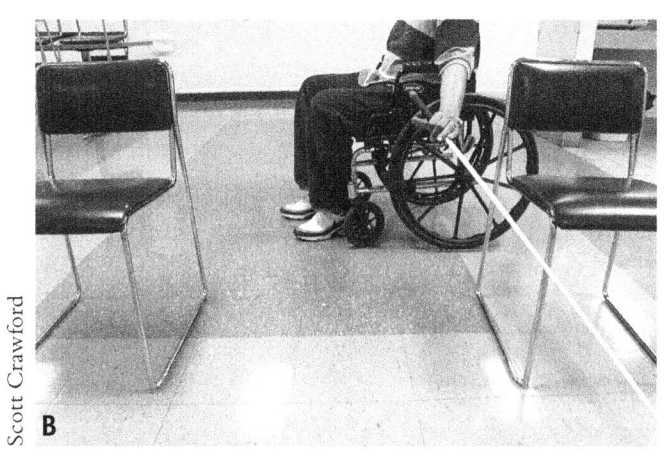

Scott Crawford

be lined up facing the opening. A scooter user may pull forward until his or her shoulder is even with the near side of the opening or his or her toes are even with the far side of the opening. The specific landmark depends on the type of chair being used and the type of turn being made.

There are six different types of turns that can be made in a wheelchair: three to the right and three to the left. A person can turn right by:

1. moving both wheels at the same time, the left forward and the right backward to create a pivot-in-place turn;

2. moving just the left wheel forward, keeping the right wheel in place, and pivoting over the right wheel; or

3. moving the right wheel backward and keeping the left wheel locked in place.

The same three possibilities are available for left turns. Different obstacles require different turns, so O&M specialists will want to teach all six types of turns to their older clients who use wheelchairs.

Carts

For many older adults, carrying objects and simultaneously utilizing a cane can be difficult or even hazardous. Some will utilize wheeled carts to transport objects such as laundry, groceries, or hot pots and pans at home or to carry large or heavy loads in the workplace (see Figure 4.22). There are several types of carts available that are suitable for this type of use. Laundry and grocery carts can have two or four wheels. Having four wheels is advantageous because it allows the cart to be pushed without being tilted onto two wheels. Some people will purchase four-wheel carts that are similar to the ones found in a workshop or warehouse. These types of carts have surfaces on which objects can be placed for transport. These carts are often helpful in kitchens and workplaces because they allow the client to carry hot or fragile items with a lower risk of bumping into other people or dropping the items.

Most cane users will pull carts instead of pushing them from behind. This allows the user to have the cane in front of the cart to clear the intended path.

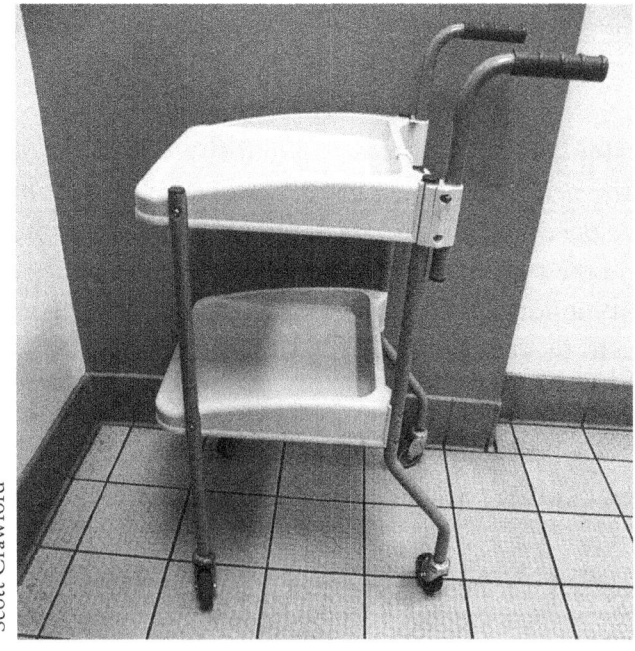

FIGURE **4.22**
Carts can provide support and assist with transporting objects.

When using a cart, clients must learn to move farther into the opening before initiating the turn or else they won't have adequate clearance.

ORIENTATION TOOLS

Tools to assist with maintaining orientation include compasses, maps, and GPS devices. Older adults can use separate specialized orientation devices or applications downloaded to smartphones. One advantage of using applications on smartphones is that clients are more likely to have them when they're needed. The disadvantage is that applications designed for the general public do not always provide an appropriate level of accessibility for people with visual impairments. New devices are constantly being developed. Consumer organizations and agencies serving people who are visually impaired are constantly reviewing new products to determine their effectiveness. (The website www.AppleVis.com; *AccessWorld* magazine, technology news for people who are blind or visually impaired from the American Foundation for the Blind; and the apps iBlink Radio and ViA are examples of the multitude of resources available that provide information on current orientation technology for people with visual impairments. For more information, see the Resources section.)

Compasses

Compasses can help older adults maintain orientation (Smith & Penrod, 2010). A compass can be used to determine direction when traveling or for maintaining line of travel while navigating open spaces such as parking lots (Crawford & Crawford, in press).

Tactile Compasses

Tactile compasses, often inaccurately called braille compasses, are specifically designed for users who are visually impaired. Tactile compasses can be worn around the neck. To use, the older adult lifts the compass and holds it flat for a few seconds before opening the lid. An individual can then feel the dial to determine in which direction north lies and then determine which direction he or she is facing. To get an accurate reading, the compass must be pointed in one direction and held steady. If the user unknowingly turns or changes the direction in which the hand is pointing, the reading will no longer be correct.

Auditory and Talking Compasses

Talking compasses are simple to use. The user points the compass forward and holds down a button (see Figure 4.23). The device then states the direction in which it is pointing. Most can identify eight different compass points. This means that the direction identified by the compass is accurate within a 45-degree range. By moving the compass back and forth to see where the compass announces a new direction, the older adult can locate the center of the range for a specific direction, which can give a more accurate reading.

Visual Compasses

Some older adults with low vision can use standard, commercially available compasses. The size of the print on the face of the compass and the visibility of the compass needle are important factors to consider when purchasing a compass for a user with low vision. Magnifiers can be used in combination with a visual compass to make the compass dial easier to read.

Smartphone Compasses

Digital compasses can provide the most accurate readings (see Figure 4.24). The digital compass that comes standard on the iPhone states the eight principal directions and provides a specific number based on 360 degrees (0 being North, 90 East, 180 South, 270 West). While having 360 separate increments may seem like a good idea, it can be very confusing to the user, since the smallest change in direction will alter the reading. For example, many students may have a difficult time figuring out what direction 112 degrees indicates. When used with VoiceOver (the iPhone's built-in screen reader), the rate of speech

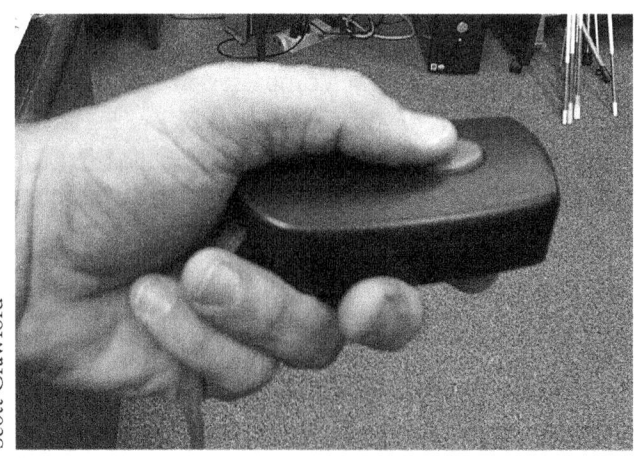

FIGURE **4.23**
Compasses can be very helpful to older adults with maintaining orientation. Talking compasses made specifically for people with visual impairments announce directions at the touch of a button.

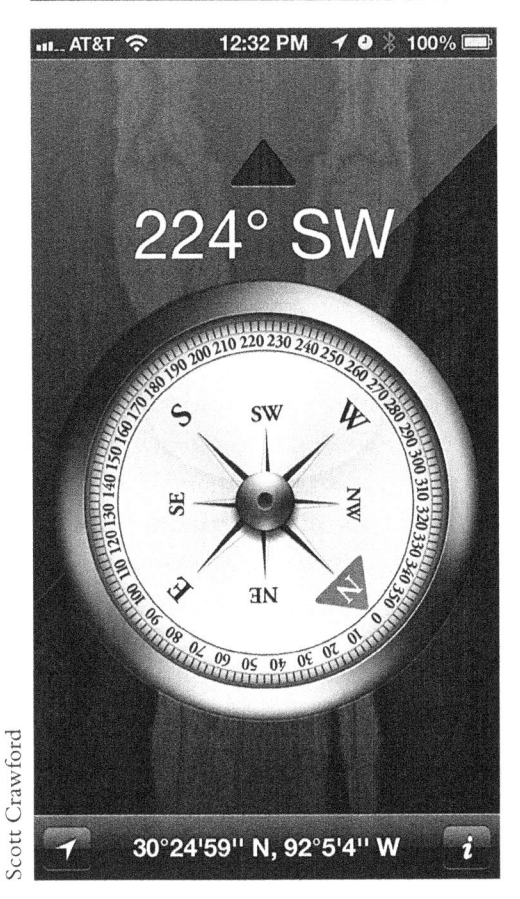

FIGURE **4.24**
Talking software makes the compasses built into smartphones accessible.

can have an effect on the accuracy of the reading. There may be significant changes in direction before the device can speak an entire reading. The faster the voice rate, the sooner the compass can correct to the new direction. The constant feedback from the application may also be distracting for some older adults. Magnets, such as those found in some phone cases and external speakers, can also affect the accuracy of the compass readings.

Global Positioning System (GPS) Receivers

GPS navigational devices are continually evolving and improving when it comes to ease of use, accuracy, and reliability. O&M specialists should not assume that older travelers will resist the use of such systems due to a fear of new technology (Smith & Penrod, 2010). A GPS device is composed of a receiver, a portable computer, and a means to relay information to the user. Not all GPS devices—and particularly not those created for people who are blind—have visual output on a screen. Some systems are extremely easy to use, with only a few buttons and limited search functions. Other systems have complex menu systems that the user must navigate (Bentzen & Marston, 2010a; Bentzen & Marston, 2010b). Familiarity with computers can be a good predictor of whether or not a given client will have success with a GPS device. If the older adult is comfortable navigating multilayer computer menus, then an advanced GPS device may be appropriate. If the older adult is more of a rote computer user, the simpler, stand-alone models will probably work best.

GPS works by triangulating the position of the user in relationship to a minimum of three satellites. A computer then takes the latitude and longitude of the receiver and plots it on maps that are loaded into the device. The higher the number of reachable satellites, and the stronger their signals, the more accurately the user's position can be determined. Satellite signals can be blocked by tall buildings, large trees, or a thick cloud cover—almost anything that might get between the satellite and the receiver. Most systems cannot be used indoors. Older adults may expect the GPS to bring them directly to the front door of a business, but commercial GPS devices are only accurate to approximately 30 feet.

Another factor that can affect accuracy is the setting of a landmark or point of interest (POI). Many GPS devices come with a variety of POIs preloaded onto their maps. The user of a GPS device can often save the locations of landmarks they prefer to use for navigation and POIs that may not be included on the preprogrammed maps. If the device was off by 30 feet when the POI was set, and then the device is 30 feet off when locating the point on a trip, it is possible the user may end up 60 feet from the desired location. Most preprogrammed POIs are set near or in the street in front of the POI. Older adults must then be able to use their mobility skills to locate the destination and complete the trip.

Standard GPS Devices

Many older adults with low vision will be able to use mainstream commercial GPS devices as long as they can read the menus and street names on the screen. The client's ability to read the screen should be tested indoors in the store before purchasing the device as well as outside in bright sunlight. Screen size of the device is one factor to consider. Larger screens may be easier to read, but may not be as easy to carry around. Small handheld units designed for hunters are usually easy to carry and are sturdier, but the screens tend to be smaller. It is helpful if the device has different modes for pedestrian and vehicle use. Some even have special modes for use on public transportation. The major disadvantage of standard GPS devices is that the menus are not voiced and most do not announce cross streets. The advantage is the lower cost and, for a user with low vision, the presence of the screen (Bentzen & Marston, 2010a; Bentzen & Marston, 2010b). Many older adults with a preference for a visual learning style will struggle with the systems designed for people who are blind because there is no screen to read.

GPS Devices Designed for People Who Are Blind

GPS devices designed specifically for use by people who are blind can be stand-alone units, or they can be add-ons to existing notetakers or computers. All of the units designed for individuals who are blind will provide accessible menus and have audio feedback about approaching cross streets (Bentzen & Marston, 2010a; Bentzen & Marston, 2010b). Many offer "bread crumb" functionality that records a user's route. The older adult can then recall the saved route whenever he or she would like to travel that way again.

Cell Phone Services

If a smart phone has text-to-speech capability, at least some aspects of a phone's built-in GPS application—or those of add-on smartphone GPS applications—will be accessible to people with visual impairments. Applications vary in price and in how much detail is provided in an accessible manner (Bentzen & Marston, 2010a; Bentzen & Marston, 2010b). An application that costs less than $2 will provide information about the nearest landmark, intersection, and address. Instead of using satellite data, some phone applications triangulate their location using cell phone towers. This allows the applications to work in conditions where the standard GPS fails. If cell service is not available, however, the location services may not work either. GPS applications also vary as to whether maps are stored on the device or accessed through the user's data plan. These factors can affect the speed and accuracy of the application, the amount of space utilized on the device, and data usage.

Maps

Visual, auditory, or tactile maps and diagrams can be very helpful for older adults learning new environments. The type that will work best for a given client depends on the complexity of the environment to be learned, the resources available, and the older adult's individual learning style. If a person who is visually impaired happens to be a visual learner, it is vital that instructional methods are adapted to help that person create an accurate mental map of the environment being learned. Tactile maps can greatly facilitate learning. For auditory learners, tactile maps may be more confusing. For them, auditory maps or auditory description in conjunction with a tactile map may be the key to success (Bentzen & Marston, 2010a; Bentzen & Marston, 2010b).

Electronic and Computer-Generated Maps

With computer programs, the Internet, and smartphones, it has never been easier for the general public to access maps. For the person with vision loss, access to these computer-generated maps may be limited (Bentzen & Marston, 2010a; Bentzen & Marston, 2010b). For clients with low vision, magnification programs may allow access. If older adults cannot see the computer screen, they may still be able to solicit sighted assistance with descriptions, access turn-by-turn directions, or print out the maps to give to drivers. Often, car, bicycle, pedestrian, or even public transportation versions of a given route are available. Some applications, such as Ariadne GPS for Apple devices, allow the user to touch a street on the screen to have the name read aloud.

Tactile Maps

Tactile maps can either be permanent, reusable diagrams or temporary kits that can be changed and reused (see Figure 4.25). However, it can be much more difficult for people who are blind to elicit information from two-dimensional tactile images than it is for sighted peers to pull information from identical visual representations (Gardner, 1996). Overly complex or detailed tactile diagrams may be difficult to understand. One advantage of several of the kits described in this section is that lines can be added one at a time, with instruction provided between each addition (Bentzen & Marston, 2010a; Bentzen & Marston, 2010b). New resources are constantly being developed, but the following are a few samples that have been effectively utilized for years (see the Resources section at the end of this book for more information on tactile graphics).

Sewell Raised Line Drawing Kit. The Sewell Raised Line Drawing Kit (see Figure 4.26) includes a rubberized clipboard and plastic sheets. When the sheets are placed on the clipboard and written on, the plastic wrinkles, creating lines that can be felt. The Sewell kit is good for simple line drawings. Lines can also be added one at a time, with instruction provided between each addition.

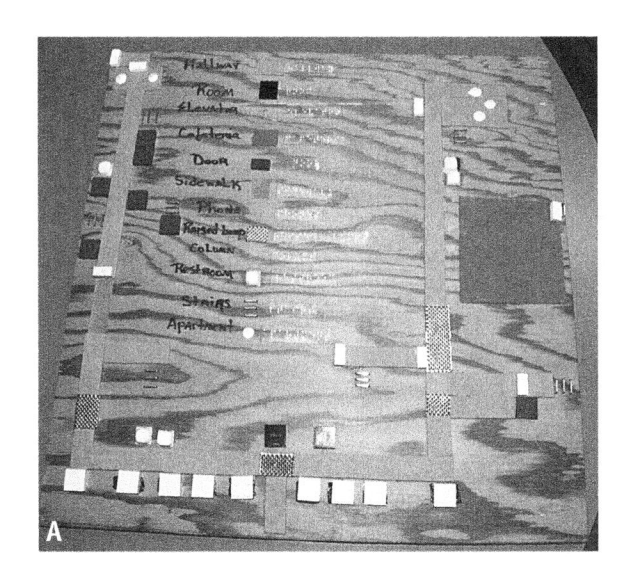

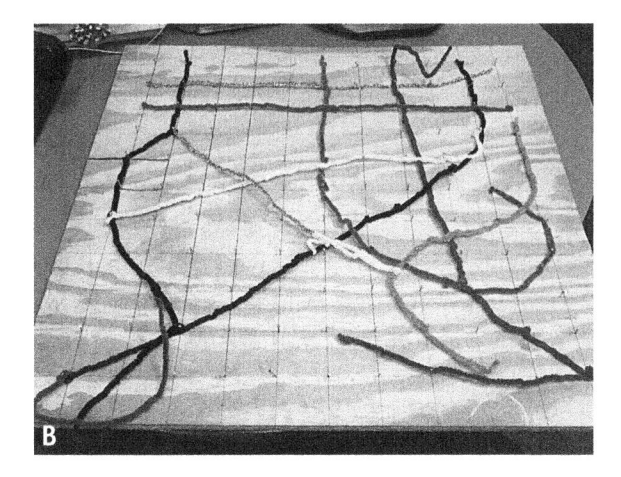

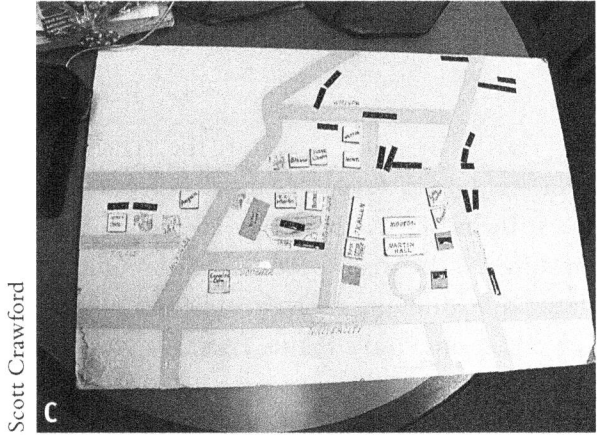

FIGURE **4.25**

Tactile maps come in a wide variety of shapes and forms. They can be permanent, temporary, or easily modified.

125

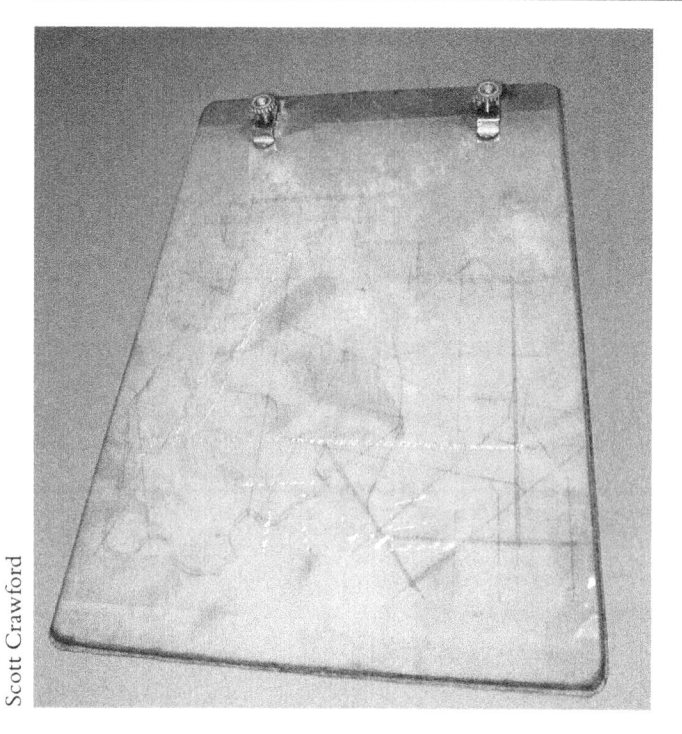

FIGURE **4.26**
When using the Sewell Raised Line Drawing Kit, any lines drawn on plastic sheets that are placed on the kit's rubberized clipboard will be raised.

Scott Crawford

Chang Tactile Graphics Kit. The Chang Tactile Graphics Kit (see Figure 4.27) includes plastic shapes with Velcro attachments that hold them in place on a felt board. The plastic pieces are yellow, providing a high degree of contrast against the black felt of the board. The kit contains squares, triangles, rectangles, strips, and pie-shaped pieces.

The Wheatley Tactile Graphics Kit. The Wheatley Tactile Graphics Kit is very similar to the Chang kit, but with a wider variety of shapes and textures that allow for greater differentiation.

APH Tactile Graphics Kit. The Tactile Graphics Kit from the American Printing House for the Blind (APH) contains a variety of tools and materials to produce custom tactile graphics, including tactile maps. It can be used with paper or thin sheets of aluminum, so the maps produced can be reused over and over again. The kit includes line-drawing tools, a rubber embossing pad, ruler, foil sheets, a braille slate and stylus, and a braille eraser, as well as a guidebook, so that different textures, shapes, and line styles can be created and braille can be added directly to the maps. The raised marks are added from

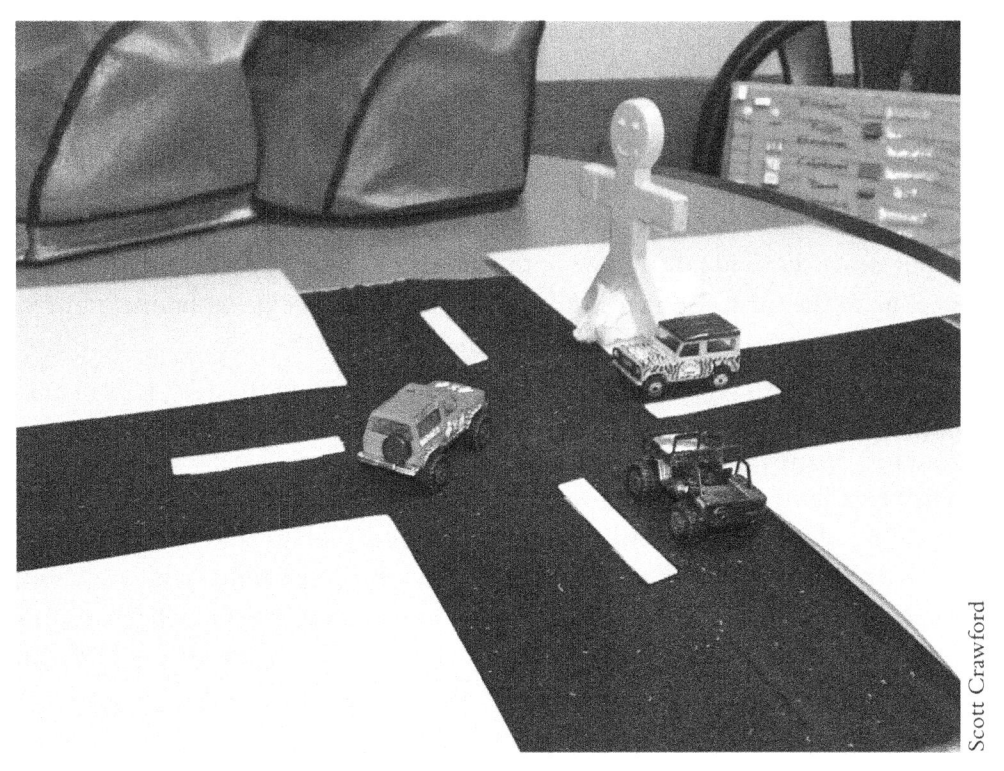

FIGURE **4.27**
The Chang Tactile Graphics Kit is a felt-covered board on which the user can attach a wide variety of yellow shapes.

the back of the sheet, so they must be drawn in mirror image to get the desired end result.

Thermoform. Thermoform machines heat and vacuum-seal plastic sheets onto master forms. Once the plastic cools it holds the shape of the master form. An unlimited number of copies can be created from one master form.

Swell Paper and Fuser. There are two types of swell paper (also known as capsule paper). One type absorbs the liquid from special pens and swells to create raised markings. The second type swells when heat is applied. Examples include the Thermo-Pen or Tactile Image Enhancer (Presley & D'Andrea, 2009).

Graphics Mode on Braille Embosser. The graphics setting available on many braille embossers allows the user to create tactile graphics using braille dots.

The diagrams to be printed may require special software like Duxbury to be converted into a file that can be embossed.

Flip Maps

Flip maps or flip charts are particularly useful for individuals who may have trouble remembering routes or procedures. In a flip map, each step of a route is put on an individual page or note card. As an older adult completes each step, he or she turns to the next card. Each card may use print, braille, figures, graphics, or a combination of these elements.

Auditory Maps

Auditory maps are basically systematic verbal descriptions of an environment. They can be recorded, typed out, or spoken directly from the O&M specialist to the older adult. Another option for auditory maps is available through many of the GPS devices designed specifically for older adults who are blind. Many have a setting that announces the sequences of streets. When practicing or familiarizing him- or herself with an environment, the older adult can make a virtual "turn" and travel in any desired direction.

Communication Devices

Older adults who struggle with communicating with the general public can be assisted by wide a variety of products that are commercially available or that can be created by the people who need them. These devices can assist with both expressive and receptive communication. All travelers should be able to utilize a variety of different communication strategies and aids when out in the environment, as different situations will require different tools (Bourquin & Sauerburger, 2005).

Communication Cards and Signs

Bourquin and Sauerburger (2005) specified that for communication cards to be effective, they must follow a specific sequence. (See Sauerburger's website, www.sauerburger.org, for more information.) First, the card should list exactly what the person wants to communicate (CROSS the STREET, TAKE Me to the CASHIER, TAKE Me to the EXIT, and so on). Second, the card should list what the reader can do to acknowledge that he or she is willing to help the older adult (TAP my SHOULDER if you can help). Finally, the card can state the person's disability or explain why the person needs assistance (Sauerburger, 1993; Sauerburger & Jones, 1997). Photo albums and ring binders can be used to assist with organization of an individual's cards and signs (see Figure 4.28 for examples of various communication signs). While often associated with deafblind travelers—those who have both hearing and vision impairments—communication cards and signs can assist any traveler with soliciting assistance. Communication signs are usually made large enough for passing motorists to read, greatly increasing the pool of possible people who can assist the older adult.

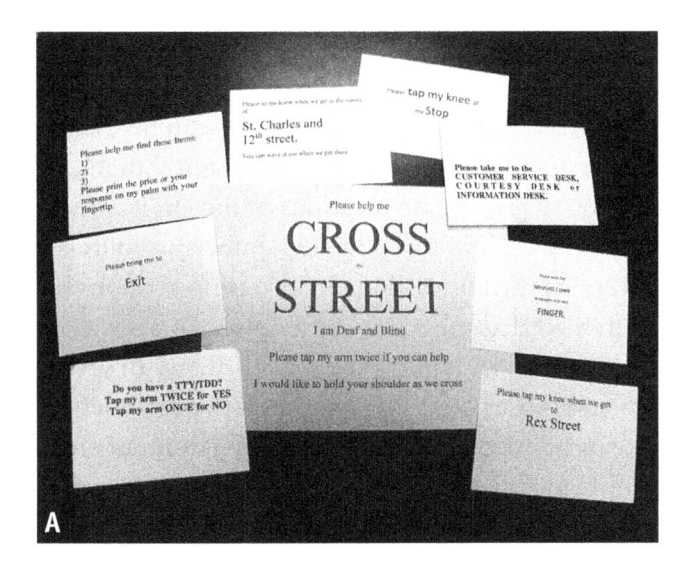

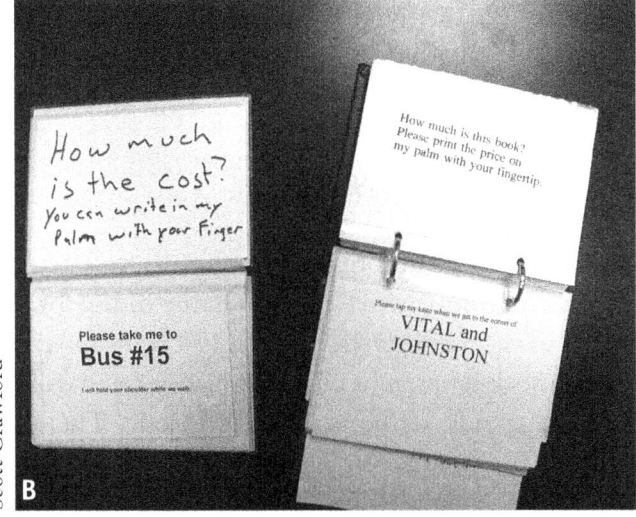

FIGURE **4.28**
Communication cards and signs are frequently used by people who are deafblind, but they can also solicit assistance for any person who is visually impaired.

Pads and Markers

For older adults who may have problems with hearing or with speaking loud enough, a simple pad and felt-tip marker can be invaluable. The pad may be used for either expressive or receptive communication. To use the pad for soliciting assistance, older adults should write their primary needs in large print and note less essential information in smaller print. This focuses the passing person's attention on what the older adult wants and increases the chances that the potential helper will stop. Notes written on yellow paper may be easier for older adults with low vision to read than notes written on white paper (Sauerburger, 1993).

Audio Recorders

For many older adults, audio recorders can be an effective memory device that can also assist with expressive communication. Recorders can be used to remember phone numbers, addresses, step-by-step route directions, bus schedules and route information, audio maps, and descriptions of the environment to be traveled. Some older adults have a difficult time remembering addresses or destinations to give to drivers. Some forget vital pieces of information that need to be communicated. Prerecorded messages can be used to assist with communication with other people. Older adults who have issues with speaking loudly enough or clearly enough to be understood can use recorders to relay information. Messages can be prerecorded by the user in a quiet environment, or by friends and family members for the older adult to use as needed.

Voice Amplifiers

Another alternative for older adults with a soft voice is to utilize voice amplifiers. When using an amplifier, the older adult speaks into a microphone and the amplified voice is transmitted by a speaker. Volume controls adjust the sound for a variety of environments.

Assistive Listening Devices

Many older adults need to utilize hearing aids or other amplification systems to access information from their environments. These can come in the form of wired headphones connected to receiving microphones, FM transmitters, Bluetooth amplification systems, neck loops, and others. Some systems work in conjunction with a user's hearing aids, while others stand alone. The effectiveness of each device depends on the type of hearing loss, ambient noise level in the environment, and sound source. Compatibility between devices is an important factor in selecting assistive listening devices. Maintenance is another key issue, as ear wax can block tubes and batteries can be low on power or dead. Older adults may want to carry spare backup batteries (see Chapter 2 for more information on hearing loss and hearing aids).

Low Vision Devices Used for O&M

Older adults with vision loss benefit from the use of low vision devices—also referred to as optical devices—when traveling (see Figure 4.29). These devices are prescribed by low vision specialists (Geruschat & Smith, 2010).

Monocular Telescopes

Monocular telescopes can be either handheld or mounted to eyeglasses. Most, but not all, are focusable. The end that is held closer to the eye holds the ocular

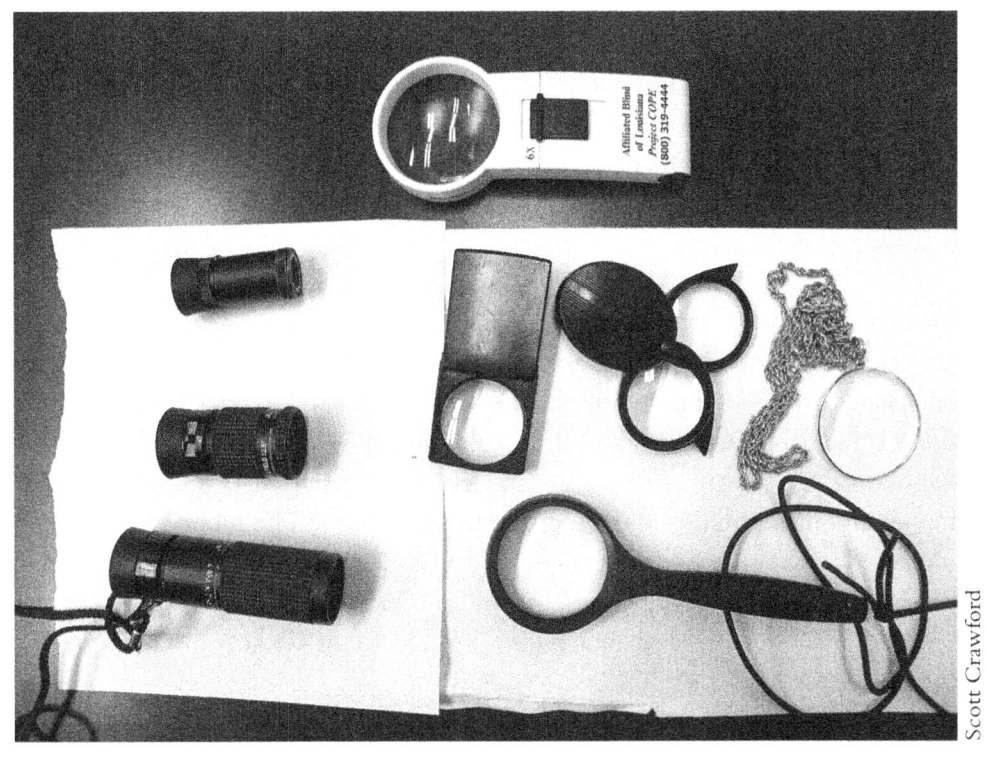

FIGURE **4.29**

Low vision devices such as those pictured here can be used to assist with reading signage, maps, directions, and transportation schedules. Monocular telescopes are pictured on the left, and magnifiers are shown at the top and right.

lens. The end pointed at the target holds the objective lens. The device can be reversed to get a minimized view of the target. Most people do not find such minification to be helpful, but for a few older adults with reduced visual fields, minification can assist with spotting a target.

The strength of most monocular telescopes is described with the amount of magnification listed first—such as 4X, 6X, or 8X—and the diameter of the lens (measured in millimeters) listed second—such as 4X×16, 8X×30. The larger the first number, the greater the magnification. The larger the second number, the larger the field of view and the greater the amount of light gathering, which brightens the image. Some monocular telescopes are listed as being extra-close focus. This designation means that an individual can focus on an object 1 to 2 feet in front of the lens instead of the standard minimum distance of around 8 to 10 feet. See Sidebar 4.4 for some suggestions for training clients in the use of monoculars.

Binoculars

For distance viewing, binoculars, which have a lens for each eye, are often easier to use than monocular telescopes, as their design makes it easier to hold them in line with the line of sight. People who struggle with spotting through monocular telescopes may be more successful with binoculars. Focusing may be easier as well.

Bioptics

Bioptics are telescopes that are mounted onto the lenses of eyeglasses. The telescopes are used for distance reading tasks and the carrier lens holds the user's standard prescription for distance viewing. The advantage of bioptics is hands-free use. In most cases, the devices are smaller than monocular telescopes and have smaller diameters and fields of view. The telescope is usually mounted in the superior (upper) field of vision. The user typically has to tilt the head slightly to bring the telescope in line with the visual target. Some bioptics are focusable, but many have a fixed focus set at a distance greater than 20 feet.

Handheld Magnifiers

Many older adults have a variety of magnifiers that meet specific needs. For instance, a client may have a larger electronic desktop magnifier at home and a smaller pocket or pendant magnifier for travel.

SIDEBAR 4.4

Training Clients to Use Distance Devices

Distance devices for the purposes of this sidebar include monocular telescopes, binoculars, and bioptics. The strategies described here can be used for any of these types of distance magnification devices. The steps presented here use a simple to complex approach. Each skill builds on the previous one. Once the older adult understands each of the strategies, they can be integrated and the device used to its fullest potential. The O&M specialist will want to cover the following tasks when teaching older clients to use distance devices.

ALIGNMENT

To successfully utilize most of the distance devices, the tube of the device must be in line with the older adult's best vision and the visual target. If a client complains that all he or she sees is black, the client is probably holding the device out of alignment with the line of sight. If the tube of the device does not point straight out from the eye, the client may only see the side of the tube. For some clients, successfully using the device may involve the use of eccentric viewing.

To help older clients learn to hold a distance device straight, turn off all the lights in the room, hold a light to the objective end (farthest from the eye), and have the client look for the light. He or she may need to move the device up and down or side to side until he or she spots the light. The light should not be so bright that it hurts the client to look at it.

PREFOCUSING

To teach the use of a monocular telescope, begin by having the client prefocus the telescope (if the monocular does not have autofocus). For objects in the distance, the monocular should be shortened as much as possible. For closer objects, the device needs to be lengthened as much as possible. With practice, older adults may be able to adjust the device to points in between those two extremes based on the distance to the target. Once the monocular is prefocused, the client may fix his or her gaze on the object and then bring the telescope up to the eye. Once the object is in view through the telescope, the client can refine the focus of the device by first adjusting the focus until he or she thinks it is clear, and then going just past that point to make sure there is no more room for improvement.

(continued)

SIDEBAR 4.4 (*continued*)

SPOTTING

The skill of spotting involves using the distance device to locate a specific target such as a sign or pole. Systematic scanning patterns may be needed to locate targets against a visually complex background.

When teaching spotting, first have the client look in the general direction of the target without the monocular. Next, have the client bring the monocular up to the eye in line with the target. Once in the general area of the target, the older adult should use a systematic search pattern to hone in on the specific target. Examples of systematic search patterns include circular or grid patterns. Circular patterns consist of the user moving the monocular in very small circles and gradually increasing the size of the circle until the target is located. In grid patterns, the client's gaze is moved back and forth across the target area, slightly shifting the line of sight with each pass. If the target is not found moving side to side, the user then recovers the target area moving the gaze up and down. With either pattern, overlapping "strokes" should be used so that the target is not missed because it is between two passes.

TRACING

Tracing involves following the course or shape of something—such as a pole, the roofline of a house, text in a book, edge of a door, or similar feature—in the environment with the distance device. Tracing is a good strategy to simplify a complex environment and locate the desired sign or part of the environment needed for orientation. The same strategy is used in near work when the older adult struggles to follow a line of letters or words while using a magnifier.

TRACKING

Tracking is more complex and involves maintaining focus on a moving target (like a bus) when the viewer is stationary, or maintaining focus on a stationary target while the viewer is moving (such as looking at a building while riding in a car). Looking through a device while walking should be discouraged, as doing so can lead to accidents. The older adult should stop, complete his or her reading task (for example, reading the street sign or a building name), and then continue moving.

REDUCING SHAKE

Telescopes magnify hand movement to the same degree that they magnify objects. Especially with higher strength magnifiers, a user's hand movement may make the viewing area shake too much to allow for efficient reading.

> To reduce movement, once the client has focused the device, the hand holding the device can be steadied by the opposite hand. The arms can then be pulled tight to the torso. This positioning assists with maintaining a steadier image. Alternatively, the client can brace the hand holding the telescope on a stationary object, resting the elbow on the opposite forearm or hugging the elbow of the arm holding the magnifier to the torso with the opposite hand (Pogrund et al., 2012).

Portable magnifiers can be a valuable resource while traveling. They can be used to read directions, maps, bus schedules, addresses, phone numbers, or phone screens. Portable magnifiers should be small enough that they are easy to access, store, and transport, yet large enough for efficient use.

Handheld electronic magnification systems (video magnifiers) can assist with O&M either at home in the route-planning process or in the community to spot landmarks or to read signs and maps. Some electronic magnifier screens are very difficult to read in bright sunlight without shading the screen somehow. Units that include a freeze mode allow the older adult to hold the device up to a shelf, sign, or other target not at eye level, freeze the image, and then bring the magnifier up to the eyes for reading.

Cameras and Video Cameras

As an alternative to specialized devices, some older adults can use zoom-enabled still or video cameras for magnification. However, there is a significant difference in quality between optical and digital zoom. Optical zoom, which is accomplished by adjusting lenses, does not degrade the quality of the image. With most digital zoom features, the more magnified the image becomes, the more pixelated it will appear. Individuals will have to determine what is most important for them, size or clarity. Some older adults will prefer large liquid-crystal display (LCD) or light-emitting diode (LED) screens, but these can be difficult to see, especially outdoors in bright light. For these users, cameras with optical viewfinders (eyepieces) may be more effective. Most digital cameras and camera phones can zoom in on a saved still photo (as opposed to zooming in on an object and then taking the photo). By taking the photo with lower or no magnification, the amount of blurring caused by hand shaking is reduced, which can improve the quality of the image overall. Tripods or monopods can also be used to increase image quality by reducing camera shake.

Sunwear and Glare Reduction

The use of appropriate sunwear (such as absorptive or tinted lenses) can greatly facilitate travel for most older adults with low vision (Geruschat & Smith, 2010). Sunglasses appropriately matched to the user's needs can reduce glare, increase contrast, and reduce eye pain and strain. As a result, sunglasses can increase the amount of visual information received by the older adult. Even older adults with little or no usable vision can benefit from the use of sunglasses. The lenses can act as a barrier to low branches or other debris that may be stirred up into the air. It is important that the older adult be allowed to compare the various sunglass grades, opacities, and tints in bright sunlight, shade, and in overcast conditions. The tint that is most effective may vary depending on the conditions present on any given day. O&M specialists will want to ask the older adult which pair allows him or her to see more clearly. In addition, O&M specialists should prompt the client to view all elements in the environment through each pair of sunglasses. Using questions such as "Which one lets you see the edge of the sidewalk?" "Which one lets you see the farthest into the distance?" and "Which one soothes your eyes most?" can guide the client to evaluate the usefulness of the lenses under consideration. Often, older adults will initially pick the pair that does the best job of blocking light. This may lead to having a lens that is too dark and causes the older adult to miss cracks and drop-offs, and to drift off the edge of the sidewalk.

Lens Tints. While many low vision specialists will recommend specific tints based on an older adult's visual diagnosis, it is best to give the older adult the opportunity to determine the specific tint that is most effective for him or her. Often, older adults with age-related macular degeneration may have a preference for gray or blue-gray tints, and older adults with retinitis pigmentosa may prefer a shade of amber. Sunglasses are available in a myriad of other colors including smoke, plum, yellow, green, orange, and red, to name just a few. Sunglass lenses can also block infrared, ultraviolet, or blue light, and can reduce glare. Each of these types of lenses will alter the wearer's vision in a different way.

Opacity. Most types of sunglasses will specify lens opacity by stating the percentage of visible light that is allowed to pass through the lens; the smaller the indicated percentage, the darker the lens. Many older adults with low vision will switch among multiple pairs of sunglasses with different opacities as lighting conditions change. They may have one pair for bright sunny days, a second pair for overcast days, and a third pair for indoor use. Some older adults will wear multiple pairs of glasses that can be quickly switched or recombined as lighting changes. Sunglasses with lightly tinted (low opacity) lenses can greatly reduce glare or eye strain from overhead florescent lighting, computer screens, or sunlight coming through windows.

Frame Style. Frames for sunglasses come in a variety of styles including some that will fit over existing prescription eyeglasses. These sunglasses rest over the top of the older adult's spectacles and come all the way to the forehead. For people who do not wear prescription eyeglasses, blade-style lenses that wrap around the side of the face and come up to the forehead are most effective at reducing glare without distorting the view through the sides of the sunglasses.

Some older adults have used sunglasses to help their eyes adapt to lighting changes. One person stated that when he tried to locate objects on a shelf, he would put on his sunglasses, leave them on for a few seconds, and when he took them off, he could see what was on the shelf more clearly. By putting on the sunglasses, he forced his pupils to dilate. When he then took the sunglasses off, more light was reaching his retina, allowing him to see more of what was on the shelf.

SUMMARY

A wide and ever-changing array of tools is available to assist older adults with O&M training. It is recommended that the O&M specialist keep an open mind when it comes to the devices, technologies, and techniques that may help an older client. Selection should include consultation among the O&M specialist, other appropriate medical professionals, and the client. Not every older adult will be able to safely or effectively use every tool or technique; strategies will need to be adapted to the abilities and needs of each client.

Effective collaboration among team members is necessary to ensure the prescription of the most effective tools and training. Recommended travel devices—including cane type, length, and tip—will depend on the physical abilities, purpose of travel, travel environment, and personal preference of each client. Orthopedic devices require consultation with other medical professionals, including occupational and physical therapists. It is sometimes assumed that people with visual impairments cannot independently utilize orthopedic devices, especially motorized ones, but with instruction from qualified specialists and modification of techniques as necessary, many older adults with vision loss learn to be safe and effective using these tools. Older adults who have had little or no instruction, or who are using devices that have been inherited or donated without being sized or set properly, can experience difficulties.

To have the best chance at effective O&M, older adults will need to have a variety of tools at their disposal. O&M specialists will want to expose their clients to as many options as possible and to assess which tools work best for each client. The tools selected must meet the unique characteristics of each individual. To ensure safety and optimum success for the older adult, O&M specialists should consult with professionals who specialize in the selected tools. Occupational therapists, physical therapists, low vision therapists, vision rehabilitation therapists, assistive technology O&M specialists, and other specialists can all play a vital role in successful O&M training.

LEARNING ACTIVITIES

1. Find a variety of mobility devices (such as a walker, support cane, and wheelchair) and try some of the techniques outlined in this chapter. Do not simulate a visual impairment unless you have a partner to ensure your safety.
2. Visit an assisted living facility and, in a 1–2 page report, note the different mobility tools used by the residents.
3. Go to an outdoor goods store to see which retail products can be used by older people with vision loss to improve their O&M skills.
4. Perform a search on a smartphone for applications related to the terms "blind," "low vision," and "deaf" to see the types of applications available to people with vision loss and hearing impairments.

References

Bentzen, B. L., & Marston, J. R. (2010a). Orientation aids for students with vision loss. In W. R. Wiener, R. L. Welsh, & B. B. Blasch (Eds.), *Foundations of orientation and mobility: Vol. I. History and theory* (3rd ed., pp. 296–323). New York: AFB Press.

Bentzen, B. L., & Marston, J. R. (2010b). Teaching the use of orientation aids for orientation and mobility. In W. R. Wiener, R. L. Welsh, & B. B. Blasch

(Eds.), *Foundations of orientation and mobility: Vol. II. Instructional strategies and practical applications* (3rd ed., pp. 315–351). New York: AFB Press.

Bourquin, E., & Sauerburger, D. (2005). Teaching deaf-blind people to communicate and interact with the public: Critical issues for travelers who are deaf-blind. *RE:view, 37*(3), 109–116.

Crawford, J. S., & Crawford, P. (in press). *Orientation and mobility for wheelchair users.* Louisville, KY: American Printing House for the Blind.

Franck, L., Haneline, R., Brooks, A., & Whitstock, R. (2010). Dog guides for orientation and mobility. In W. R. Wiener, R. L. Welsh, & B. B. Blasch (Eds.), *Foundations of orientation and mobility: Vol. I. History and theory* (3rd ed., pp. 277–295). New York: AFB Press.

Gardner, J. A. (1996). Tactile graphics, an overview and resource guide. *Information Technology and Disabilities E-Journal, 3*(4).

Geruschat, D. R., & Smith, A. J. (2010). Low vision for orientation and mobility. In W. R. Wiener, R. L. Welsh, & B. B. Blasch (Eds.), *Foundations of orientation and mobility: Vol. I. History and theory* (3rd ed., pp. 63–83). New York: AFB Press.

Ivanchenko, V., Coughlan, J., Gerrey, W., & Shen, H. (2008, October). *Computer vision-based clear path guidance for blind wheelchair users.* Paper presented at the 10th International ACM SIGACCESS Conference on Computers and Accessibility, Halifax, Nova Scotia, Canada.

Jacobson, W. H. (2013). *The art and science of teaching orientation and mobility to persons with visual impairment.* New York: AFB Press.

Pogrund, R., Sewell, D., Anderson, H., Calaci, L., Cowart, M. F., Gonzalez, C. M., . . . Roberson-Smith, B. (2012). *Teaching age-appropriate purposeful skills (TAPS): An orientation and mobility curriculum for students with visual impairments* (3rd ed.). Austin: Texas School for the Blind and Visually Impaired.

Presley, I., & D'Andrea, F. M. (2009). *Assitive technology for students who are blind or visually impaired: A guide to assessment.* New York: AFB Press.

Rosen, S., & Crawford, J. S. (2010). Teaching orientation and mobility to learners with visual, physical, and health impairments. In W. R. Wiener, R. L. Welsh, & B. B. Blasch (Eds.), *Foundations of orientation and mobility: Vol. II. Instructional strategies and practical applications* (3rd ed., pp. 564–623). New York: AFB Press.

Sauerburger, D. (1993). *Independence without sight or sound: Suggestions for practitioners working with deaf-blind adults.* New York: AFB Press.

Sauerburger, D., & Jones, S. (1997). Corner to corner: How can deaf-blind travelers solicit aid effectively? *RE:view, 29*(1), 34–44.

Smith, D. L., & Penrod, W. M. (2010). Adaptive technology for orientation and mobility. In W. R. Wiener, R. L. Welsh, & B. B. Blasch (Eds.), *Foundations of orientation and mobility: Vol. I. History and theory* (3rd ed., pp. 241–276). New York: AFB Press.

CHAPTER 5

Environmental Adaptation and Modification
Pat Crawford and Laura Bozeman

Many people modify their environments without consciously thinking about it. Moving a chair to face a friend during a conversation is considered polite and also helps with hearing by allowing for increased access to visual and auditory clues. Angling a chair away from the window to read a book can be an intuitive response for increasing reading comfort and reducing glare on the page. Pushing a dining chair under the table may be a habit learned in childhood because it keeps a clear pathway for grandma or prevents small children from climbing. Most people are good at modifying the environment to meet their needs.

Another way people respond to the environment is to adapt by changing their approach or personal behavior. Turning one's head to funnel sound to an ear, navigating along the outside edge of a sidewalk to avoid overhanging branches or shrubs, or organizing a shopping list by how items are grouped in the store for more efficient travel are examples of how people adapt to the environment.

What happens when the subconscious, intuitive, or personal habits of adapting and modifying the environment no longer meet day-to-day needs? How can an orientation and mobility (O&M) specialist help his or her clients figure out what works best for them? An underlying premise of this chapter is that adaptive and modified solutions are highly individualized and contextually specific to a particular environment, the desired outcome, and personal abilities. This chapter presents a process (see Figure 5.1) for bringing creative problem-solving skills to the forefront to assist the O&M specialist in the dissection, analysis, and reconceptualization of a clients' environment and behaviors.

The first step in the process of evaluating the client's surroundings is to understand why the built environment is the way it is. An overview of the

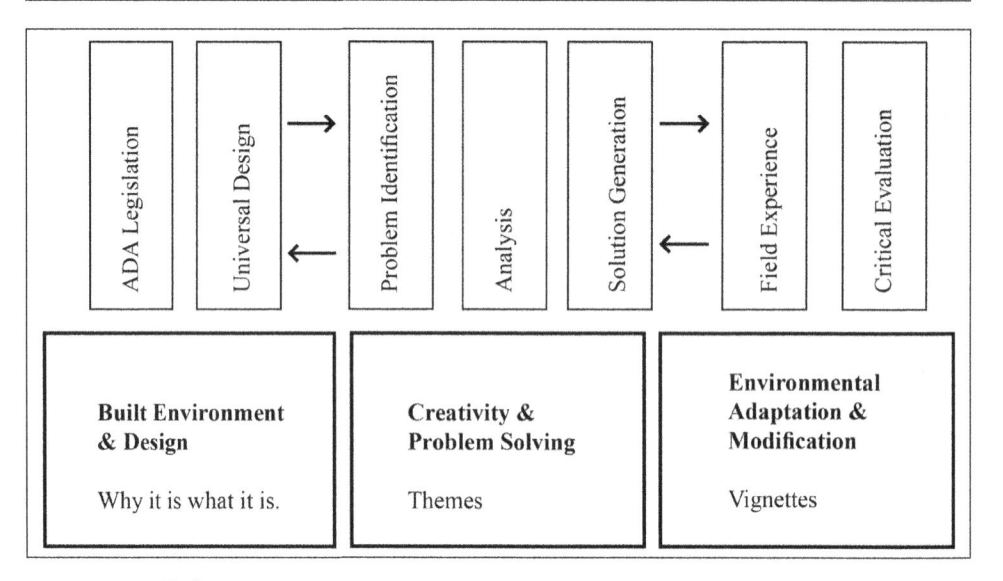

FIGURE 5.1
Analysis Process
Overview of the process for analyzing the built environment, problem solving, and generating solutions for environmental adaptation and modification.

1990 Americans with Disabilities Act (ADA) and universal design provide the framework for analyzing existing conditions and learning from what others have done. An understanding of why (or why not) things are built in certain ways to meet federal regulations or design principles assists with exploring new solutions.

The second step is activating creative and problem-solving processes to explore potential solutions that are truly specific to an individual's needs. One way to enhance creativity is to look at a problem from multiple perspectives. To that end, this chapter represents diverse perspectives and areas of expertise—O&M, vision rehabilitation therapy, and education—on the design and construction of accessible environments and the development of accessibility policy. Integrating these perspectives allows a broad, interconnected approach to the issues.

This chapter looks at the third step of analysis and idea-generating processes through a number of themes: consistency, contrast, texture, and transitions, and is based on an analysis of a variety of actual field experiences with clients. Vignettes are used to model the process of identifying problems, generating solutions, and applying themes. The goal is for O&M specialists to be able to apply the process to each individual client's situation.

Older adults may have a variety of health issues that impact function and require additional members on the team. For the older adult with balance issues, for example, the physical therapist is a necessary component of the individual's plan of support and training. For the older adult with hearing loss and hearing aids, the audiologist may be a critical member of the team. Other members include rehabilitation counselors, social workers, and occupational therapists who share the goal to support the client's independence and interests. Integrated plans of support from the team of professionals can improve the outcomes for the older individual with visual impairment (Griffin-Shirley & Welsh, 2010). The older adult as well as the O&M specialist can benefit from the collective approach to assessing the environment for safety and function.

THE BUILT ENVIRONMENT AND DESIGN
Built Environment

The built environment, as distinguished from the natural environment, is the physical space built by humans for life, work, education, and play. Examples include buildings, cities, urban spaces, walkways, and streets.

Americans with Disabilities Act

The 1990 Americans with Disabilities Act (P.L. 101–336) was passed to prohibit discrimination against people with disabilities in employment, transportation, public accommodation, communications, and governmental activities; as such, its implementation is widely concerned with ensuring that the built environment is accessible to people with disabilities. The spirit of the act is to provide equal access and opportunity for all (Outdoor Developed Areas Regulatory Negotiation Committee of the U.S. Access Board, personal communication, 2007). The law itself is broad and intended to create an environment in which people can find the most effective and creative ways for everyone to participate and contribute to society, with fair expectations of accommodation for users as well as providers.

Compliance with the provisions of the ADA is defined and measured, in a legal sense, through scoping and technical provisions provided by the Access Board, a federal agency that promotes accessibility for people with disabilities through the development of guidelines and standards. These provisions are set out in the ADA Standards for Accessible Design—the most recent of which were published in 2010 (U.S. Department of Justice, 2010a)—with detailed specifications provided in the ADA Accessibility Guidelines (U.S. Access Board, 2002). The scoping provisions delineate a minimum quantity or percentage of elements (such as restaurant menus, door signs), activity spaces (such as parking stalls or apartments), or service access points (such as window tellers or entries) that must meet the technical provisions. The technical provisions provide an "on-the-ground" measure, such as the slope of walkways (Section 401) and curb cuts (Section 406) or the size and contrast of signage (Section 701) (U.S. Department of Justice, 2010a).

ADA specifications are based on a set of standardized human dimensions and the typical skills of individuals across a range of disabilities. The definition of disability is broad, including "a physical or mental impairment that substantially limits one or more major life activities of such individual" (U.S. Equal Employment Opportunity Commission, 2008, Sec 4 [1]). The specifications are based on available research and the knowledge of experts participating in rulemaking processes, such as the Association for Blind Athletes, National Council for Independent Living, and Paralyzed Veterans of America, who served as members of the 25-person Outdoor Developed Areas Regulatory Negotiation Committee (Bradtmiller & Annis, 1997; U.S. Access Board, n.d.).

An interesting complication with the scoping and technical provisions is that what works for one person or group may not work for another; and an accessibility feature designed to accommodate a specific disability may create a barrier for another type of disability. For example, blended curbs or curb cuts that assist people who use wheelchairs and walkers by removing the barrier created by a vertical curb also remove the detectable edge or warning that would alert people with visual impairment or blindness to the transition from sidewalk to street.

The ADA does not cover every possible scenario or environment. The recommendations that do exist are often the result of extensive dialogue, testing, and retesting. Recommendations are also subject to scrutiny from many perspectives once adopted and may be further modified over time. For example, to address the hazard of blended curbs working too well (removal of the detectable edge), the 1991 Americans with Disabilities Act Accessibility Guidelines (ADAAG) required the use of truncated domes (tactile bumps) on the surface of curb cut ramps to create a detectable warning for people with visual impairments (see Figure 5.2) (U.S. Access Board, 2003).

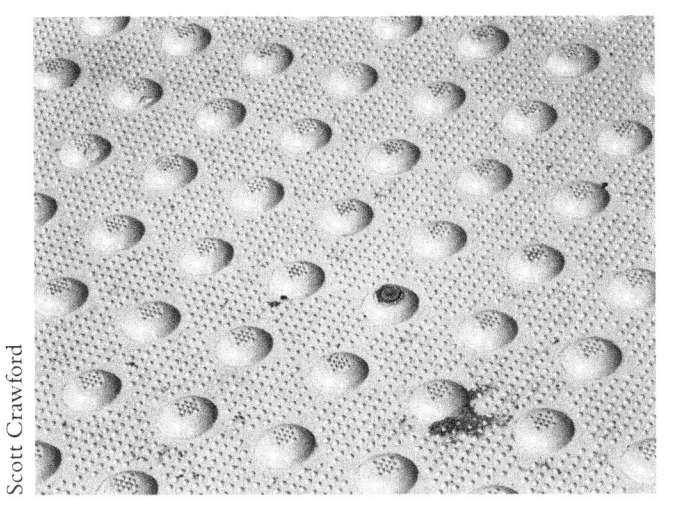

FIGURE **5.2**
Truncated domes are used internationally to indicate to people with visual impairments that they are about to leave an area of relative safety and enter an area with potential dangers such as automobiles, drop-offs, or other hazards, and when they return to a safe area.

Subsequently, truncated domes were considered to be a hazard for maneuvering wheelchairs, and the requirement was suspended from 1994 to 2001 to conduct research (U.S. Access Board, 2003). During this period, a variety of surface treatments, including horizontal grooves, exposed aggregate, and other surface patterns were tested and determined insufficient for detection of the curb cut. Truncated domes were determined to be the most effective surface treatment as a detectible and unique environmental cue for approach into the street for people with visual impairments (Barlow, Bentzen, & Franck, 2010). A modified design of the truncated domes, with more space between the domes, was endorsed by the U.S. Access Board in 2001 and became part of the required standards. The 2010 ADAAG retained the detectable warning requirement solely at transit platform edges, stating that these were the only locations where detectable warnings "significantly benefit individuals with disabilities" (U.S. Department of Justice, 2010b, Section 218). The detectable warning requirement was removed from curb ramps, hazardous vehicle areas, and reflection pools. The 2010 ADAAG technical provisions for curb ramps are detailed in Section 406. When detectable warnings (truncated domes) are provided, the technical provisions can be found in Section 705. The U.S. Access Board (2014) followed four years later with a "Detectable Warnings Update" publication. The proposed guideline requires detectable warnings at curb ramps, pedestrian islands, at-grade crossings, and unprotected boarding areas. While the guidelines are usable, they are not mandatory until implemented as standards by agencies such as the Department of Transportation and Department of Justice.

As this history illustrates, the ADAAG technical provisions are a continuous experiment in environmental adaptation and modification. It is also important to note that just because a modification or design detail is not required, that does not mean it cannot be used. ADA standards represent the minimum set of criteria. So, while scoping provisions only require detectable warnings at transit platform edges, they may also be provided in other places, such as curb ramps.

Meeting the minimum standards, in the legal language, is referred to as "accessible." Unfortunately, something that is accessible may not be usable. For example, a ramp at a maximum allowable slope of 1:12 (1 foot rise over 12 foot length) can be navigated independently by someone in a manual chair with sufficient arm strength and stamina, but not by an individual with more severe disabilities. The steepness of the slope can also be dangerous for users of electric wheelchairs with a higher center of gravity. The term "usable" can describe areas or features that are either not covered in the standards or go beyond the minimum criteria. The ADA regulations "require new facilities to be both 'accessible to' and 'usable by' people with disabilities" (Public Rights-of-Way Access Advisory Committee, 2007, p.13).

One example of an accommodation that is both accessible and usable is frequency modulation (FM) technology that picks up the voice of a speaker via a body-worn transmitter microphone. It then uses harmless radio waves to send this signal wirelessly to the listener, who wears a tiny FM receiver. The Fenway Park baseball stadium in Boston, Massachusetts, provides frequency modulation (FM) broadcasts of the live baseball game for fans with visual impairments, which makes the play-by-play accessible. To make it usable, the park offers FM receivers, free of charge, for use during the game.

Accessibility and Universal Design

In the general population, the term "accessible" is often used interchangeably with "ADA compliant." While this may be in line with the legal language, ADA compliance addresses very specific needs and issues for people with disabilities, whereas accessibility is a much broader concept. In the case of the blended curb previously described, the accommodation made traversing the curb more accessible to a wider range of the population—not just people with disabilities, but also people with strollers, wheeled cases, or carts. Accessible design can be informed by the ideas of universal design, which extends design thinking beyond people with disabilities to all people.

Universal design is design that makes products and spaces usable for the widest possible range of people. An example is the curb cut that makes navigation easier for people in wheelchairs and for people with baby strollers or rolling luggage. Much like the ADA technical requirements, when considering sidewalks, universal design looks at slope, width, height clearance, and curb cuts. But it also considers how the needs of a huge cross-section of sidewalk users can be met, including people pushing strollers, pregnant women, pairs of people who must walk side-by-side to communicate in sign language, people using umbrellas, and delivery professionals who use dollies to bring merchandise into a store.

Focusing on ADA compliance to achieve accessible design has two strong limitations. First, the government cannot mandate good design. Good design includes aesthetics, function, appropriateness for a climate or culture, or the use of creativity to solve problems. The second limitation is that the ADA standards are broad so that they can be enforced at a national scale and meet, at least minimally, the needs of people with diverse disabilities. The government cannot mandate a standard set of regulations that addresses individual needs, much less changing needs across the lifespan. O&M specialists must know these limitations of the ADA standards addressing an extensive scope in order to know how and when to pursue further modifications that may be justified for a given client.

Environmental Adaptation and Modification

Environmental adaptation and modification are where good design and individualized needs meet. Compliance with ADA can provide a framework from which to move into the finer threads of individual needs and preferences. *Environmental adaptation* is when a person changes his or her technique, process, or approach to meet his or her individual needs in the context of a specific environment. An example is navigating along the left side of a particular sidewalk to avoid the lower tree branches that encroach on the right side. Environmental modification is when a specific environment is changed to meet the needs of an individual or group. In the sidewalk example, a modification would be implementation of a tree maintenance plan to remove the branches encroaching on the sidewalk (ensuring 80-inch height clearance along the path of travel), making it safe to navigate along either side.

Individual assessment, personal skill development (adaptation), and environmental changes (modification) are explored by O&M specialists to enhance the safety and usability of an environment for a client. An O&M assessment may include some or all of the following:

- basic skills assessment
- low vision assessment
- functional needs assessment
- environmental assessment
- home, community, job, or work site assessment

These assessments look at the individual's skill level, the potential for improvement of skills, and environmental barriers. While removing or modifying an environmental barrier may improve a specific place, when individual adaptation is possible, overall independence is increased. Individual skills can be generalized across environments and situations and applied in future situations. When a specific area is modified, the modification applies to that environment alone. This is especially true where environments meet the minimum ADAAG standards for accessibility.

A *barrier* is an environmental condition that makes an activity or service inaccessible. Barriers can be classified as obstacles or hazards. An obstacle is a barrier that can be detected and avoided, such as a curb, light pole, or piece of furniture. A hazard is an environmental condition that will not be noticed or recognized using typical O&M techniques. An example of a hazard is when the open area under a staircase is not filled in or blocked (see Figure 5.3). When a person with vision loss approaches that staircase perpendicularly, a cane sweep at ground level would not detect the overhead hazard (the stairs) at head level, thus creating an unsafe condition. Placing an object such as a planter or a box under the stairway for the cane to contact can reduce the hazard.

Another example of a hazard involves integrated curbs and gutters. Integrated curb and gutter systems are created by a single pour of concrete so that there is little visual contrast to indicate the vertical edge of the curb (see Figure 5.4A), especially when viewed in bright sun or low light. For people with limited vision who do not use a cane, it can be difficult to detect the curb. Similarly, the drop-off at stair edges frequently blends in with the sidewalk as it continues away from the stairs (Figure 5.4B). Painting the riser of the curb or stair yellow and adding a 6- to 10-inch yellow stripe on the top edge of the stairs (Figure 5.4C) provides an indication that there may be a change of level.

Environmental Adaptation and Modification 149

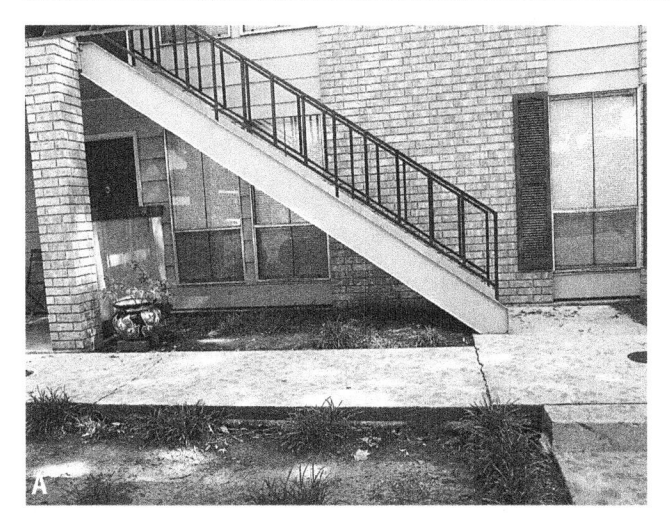

FIGURE **5.3**
The undersides of stairs can be hazardous for people with visual impairments (**A**). Using grass, planters, furniture, boxes, or railings under the stairs (**B**) can supply something for the cane to contact and reduce the hazard.

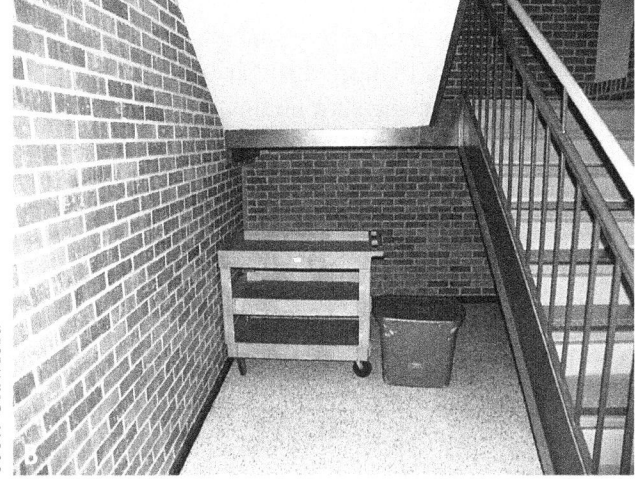

An environment can meet all the ADA requirements and still have barriers due to individual limitations. People with multiple disabilities can make access and usability even more challenging in a public environment. As noted earlier, an ADA-compliant ramp slope that uses a 1:12 ratio is accessible to most people regardless of age, mobility aid used, or gender. However, when all three factors are combined, the 1:12 ramp can be difficult to negotiate for females aged 65 and older with reduced strength or stamina, and for older adults who use wheelchairs (Sanford, Story, & Jones, 1997). If the ramp is in a residential environment or unit specifically tailored to a particular group of people, such as an assisted living center, environmental modifications might include the following:

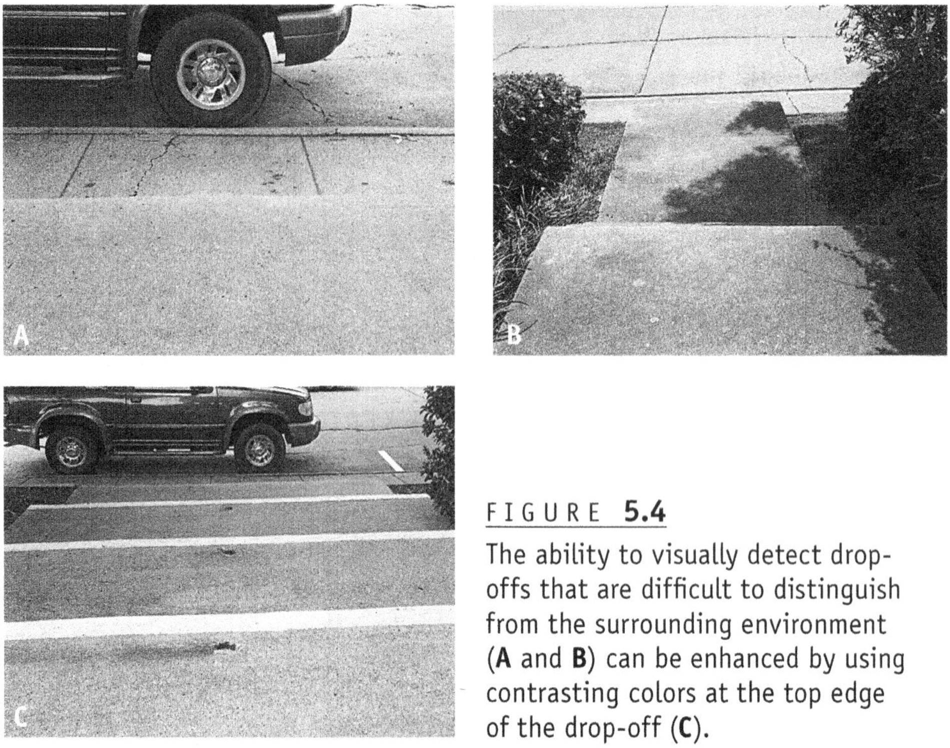

FIGURE 5.4

The ability to visually detect drop-offs that are difficult to distinguish from the surrounding environment (**A** and **B**) can be enhanced by using contrasting colors at the top edge of the drop-off (**C**).

- use a ramp with a lesser slope
- re-grade the entry if space is available, using a more accessible 1:20 (5 percent) pathway
- change the entry location
- provide a chair lift option

Adaptations could include the following:

- arrange for assistance or an aide
- switch mobility devices
- work on upper body strength training

For design professionals, builders, and O&M specialists, environmental adaptation and modification means designing the environment for flexibility in how spaces are used while also allowing for personalization. Certified aging-in-place specialists (CAPS) are part of a growing industry that specializes in residential remodeling for home modifications to support aging-in-

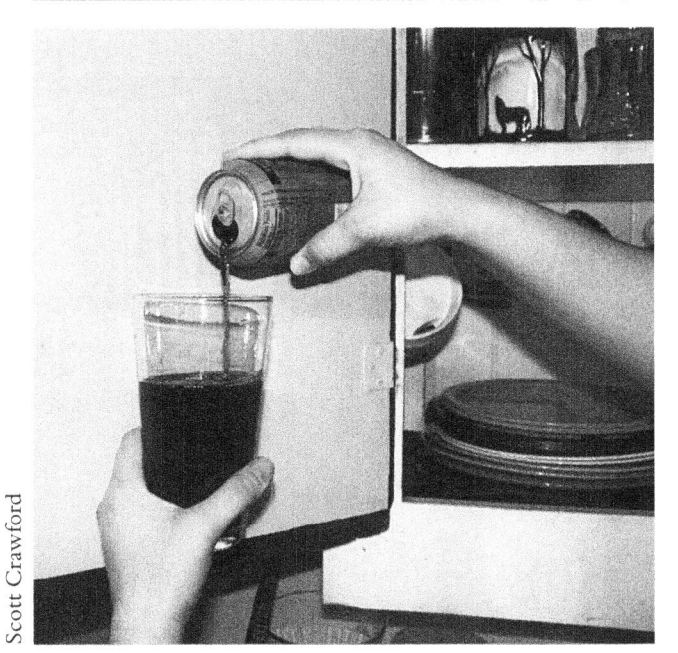

FIGURE **5.5**
Cabinet doors or counter backsplashes can be used to provide contrasting backgrounds for pouring liquids.

place (National Association of Home Builders, n.d.). Individual needs for creating an accessible environment are as unique as the individuals themselves. Finding solutions, which can often be inexpensive or easy to implement, may also mean doing or using things in nontraditional ways. Puff paint can be used to mark preferred temperature settings on stove and shower knobs. Painting the inside of cabinet doors a contrasting color to the exterior creates two surfaces, one dark and one light, that can be used as contrasting backgrounds for pouring liquids—such as milk against a dark background or a cola against a light background (see Figure 5.5). Another approach is to use light mugs for dark liquids such as coffee, and dark cups for light liquids such as milk. Cutting boards that are light on one side and dark on the other can provide contrast when cutting and chopping foods. Painting door frames a color that contrasts with the walls can also make it easier to locate doorways for a person with low vision (see Figure 5.6).

CREATIVITY AND PROBLEM SOLVING

Accessibility solutions are not always readily available, and the O&M specialist may need to take a creative approach to find the best answer for a specific situation or person. Being creative is the process of "creating original ideas

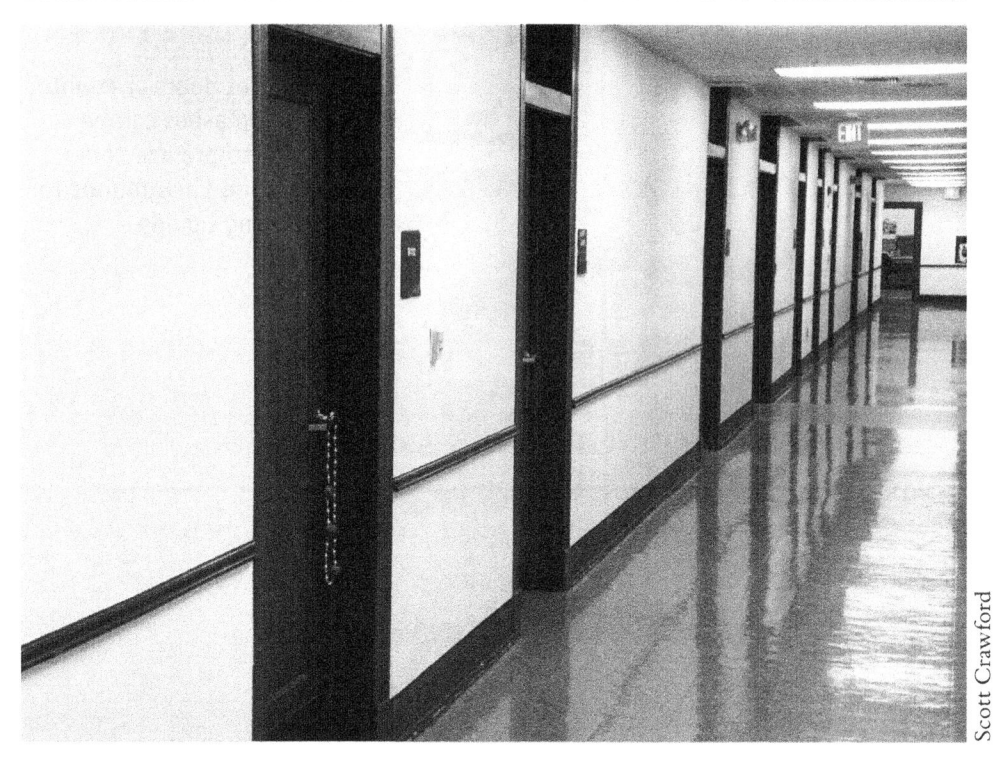

FIGURE **5.6**
Doorframes that are painted a contrasting color to the walls can be helpful in locating doorways, as can placing a specific decoration on the door handle.

that have value" (Robinson, 2011, p. 3) and are appropriate to the situation at hand. The creative process uses flexible thinking to see a problem from different perspectives and has three phases: (1) identify the problem, (2) generate solutions, and (3) evaluate critically. Creative thinking involves continually reframing the problem to reach the true essence of the issue. Detailed task analysis is vital to determining the real problem and often involves a reiterative trial-and-error process, as in the following example:

> A person living in a skilled care facility knows that his room is the seventh door down the hallway from the common room. He walks along the right (east) side of the hallway and uses hand trailing to count doors to reach his room. One day, equipment was left in the hallway and in the process of navigating around the equipment, he missed a door and ended up entering the eighth door. To address the problem, he was taught how to use O&M techniques to get around the equipment more efficiently and avoid missing

doors in his count. A secondary environmental cue, a distinctive ribbon placed around the handle on his room door, was also added to enhance orientation and recognition. The facility also initiated a new policy to help reduce the impact of equipment left in the hallway. The policy required all equipment to be stored on the left (west) side of the hallway and for all residents to use the right (east) wall for hand trailing. However, this meant that all residents were walking on the east side, regardless of which way they were walking. As with cars, putting two-way traffic in the same lane is bound to result in a few collisions. The solution was to create another policy: residents must now use their canes while navigating the hallway to provide a better preview of the environment and minimize bodily collisions.

The creative process is repetitive and moves back and forth between new ideas (divergent thinking) and refining ideas (convergent thinking) (Guilford, 1967; Michalko, 2001). When generating solutions for modifying the environment or providing an assistive device, it is helpful to think about what could be added, subtracted, modified, or used differently from its original purpose. Some examples of these types of modifications include the following:

- adding tennis balls to the legs of walkers to allow the walker to be moved without lifting
- removing the cover of the face of a clock to allow tactile exploration of the clock hand positions
- painting a cane a bright color to make it easier to locate for a person with remaining vision
- using a broom as a cane for walking in the yard to allow the user to immediately clear debris off walkways

THEMES: CONSISTENCY, CONTRAST, TEXTURE, AND TRANSITIONS

Four themes have been identified that can structure the exploration of creative solutions to vision-related barriers. The themes are consistency, contrast, texture, and transitions. The themes have both positive and negative characteristics and often occur in combination with one another.

Consistency

Consistency, in a positive sense, refers to locating or presenting information, controls, objects, and environmental cues in a similar place and manner throughout the environment. Consistency allows the O&M client to anticipate where information, a control, or object can be found. Patterns of repetitive objects can be used as navigation guides. For example, an individual with low vision or light projection could follow ceiling lights set in a grid across a cafeteria (see Figure 5.7; it is important to make sure tables and other objects are not in the line of travel indicated by the overhead light fixtures).

The O&M specialist can also consider how change in a pattern can indicate a change in the environment. When a common room is connected with hallways on opposite sides of the room, the route of travel can be identified through the use of a consistent and distinct flooring surface along the hallways and on the pathway through the open common space. A similar example can be seen in some large clothing stores, where the main aisles are surfaced with tile, while the floor under the clothing racks is carpeted.

Consistency can also be a negative in the environment. For example, when there are no changes in surface to indicate a hazard or drop-off, or lack of

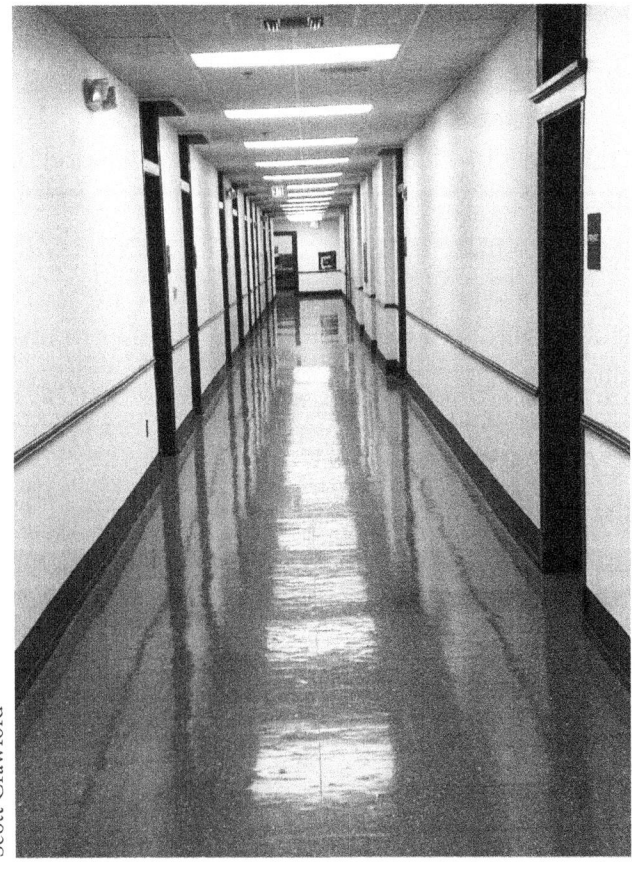

FIGURE **5.7**
The pattern of fluorescent fixtures in this corridor may help in orientation.

color differentiation in light switch plates to aid in locating them on a wall. These situations are closely aligned with contrast, which is explored next.

The following questions can be used to guide identification of problems related to consistency in the environment:

- Is something in a different location than normal or expected?
- Is something missing (such as a change in surface or color)?
- Is a cue consistently present or intermittent (such as the sound of cars, a television, or other equipment)?
- Is the same size, color, shape, or texture used for the same information or environmental cues elsewhere in the area?

Contrast

Contrast includes a visual, tactile, or auditory difference that can be used to set things apart or to signal a change in the environment. A white concrete sidewalk contrasts visually with adjoining grass or wood mulch, but blends in with white stone mulch. Using contrasting colors on doorframes, light switches, and electrical sockets may make them easier to locate (see Figure 5.8). However, the use of contrasting colors can be negated by bright sunlight or the glare of bare lightbulbs. Too much contrast can also make an environment difficult to interpret or navigate.

Uniqueness can be used judiciously as a form of contrast as well. Placing a ribbon on a doorknob or installing a wreath on a door can designate a personal room or office. Auditory signals, such unique ringtones, can be used for caller identification.

The following questions can be used to guide identification of problems related to lack of contrast in the environment:

- Is everything the same color?
- Is the lighting too bright, creating glare, or too low, reducing visual contrast?
- Are important areas or objects signaled with a detectable change?

Texture

Texture provides three-dimensional environmental information that can be detected underfoot, by a cane, or by hand. Different surface textures can reduce glare, increase traction, or change how sound travels. Braille and raised

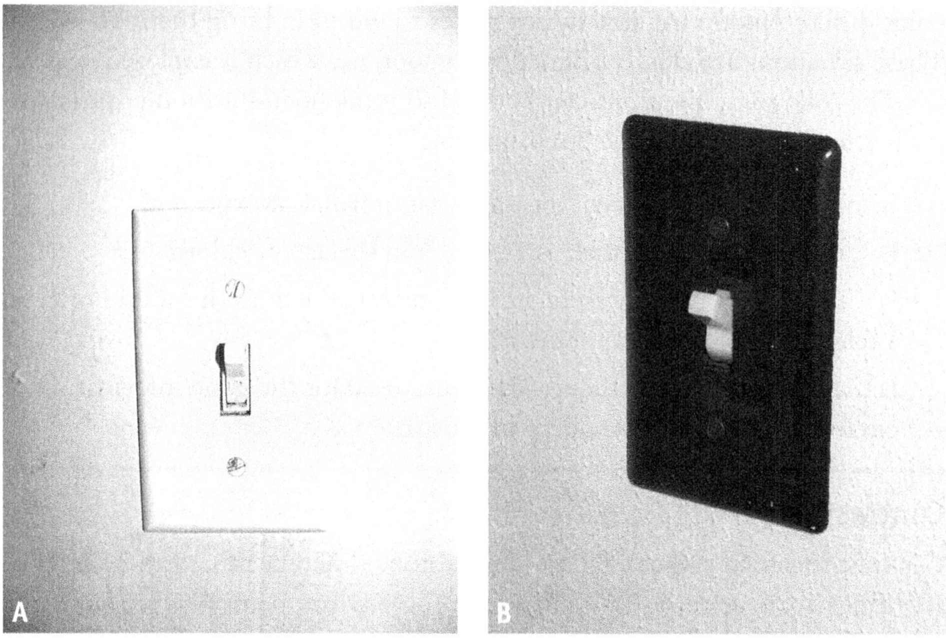

FIGURE **5.8**
Using contrasting colors for electrical outlets, light switches, and their corresponding plates can make them easier for individuals with low vision to see.

or recessed dial settings are forms of texture and serve as communication tools. A surface change from carpet to tile at the approach to stairs provides a textural cue of an environmental change.

The following questions can be used to guide identification of problems related to lack of texture in the environment:

- Does everything in the environment feel the same?
- Are important areas or edges identified with a detectable change?
- Are the raised elements detectable and within reach?

Transitions

Transitions are where materials join together or there is an important change in environment. The transition between the sidewalk and the street is an important change in materials (for example, from concrete sidewalk to blacktop) and change in environment (pedestrian to vehicular pathway). An audible walk signal indicates a transition to when it is safe to cross the street.

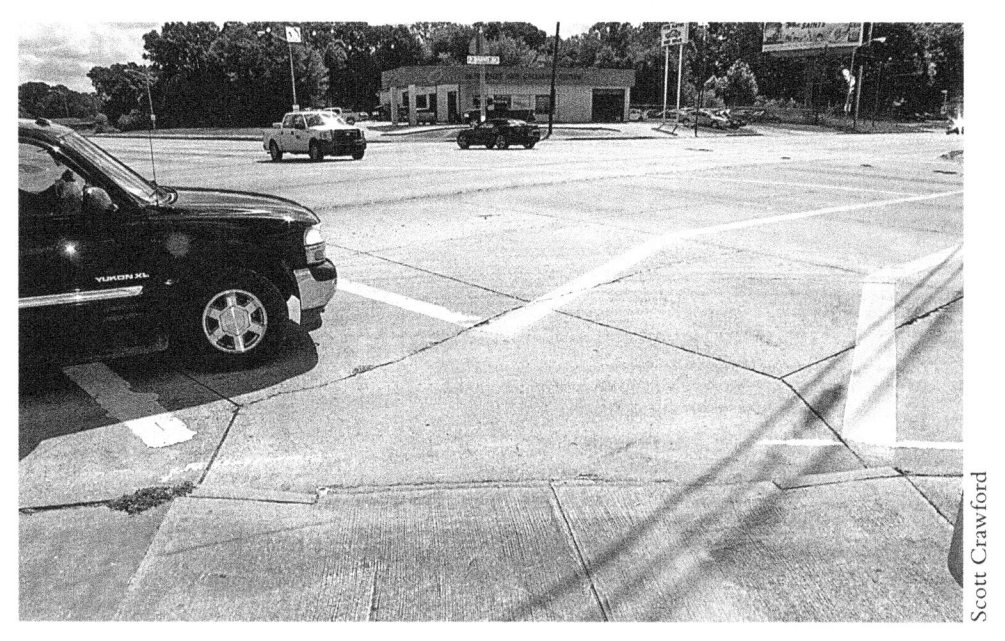

FIGURE **5.9**
Curb ramps oriented diagonally across intersections can make alignment for street crossings more difficult for travelers with visual impairments.

Sometimes a transition is identifiable but unclear. As noted earlier, a curb cut provides easier access for an individual who uses a wheelchair or walker. However, for the traveler with impaired vision to maintain orientation, the blended area needs to be aligned with the direction of the sidewalk so the person's line of travel is not interrupted. Often, to conserve costs, the curb cut or blend is oriented diagonally at the corner of the sidewalk (see Figure 5.9) rather than pointing directly into the crosswalk in both directions, so that only one cut is necessary. Following a diagonal curb cut might put a traveler into the middle of the intersection or land him or her on an unintended corner.

Blended curbs are a smooth sloping transition from a sidewalk to a vehicular or other pathway (see Figure 5.10). In these situations, a distinct textural change is needed to highlight the change from a pedestrian to a vehicular area.

The change in material between a kitchen countertop and the stovetop is an example of a boundary that can increase safety. An example of environmental transition on a micro scale is the change between the heat settings on a stove dial.

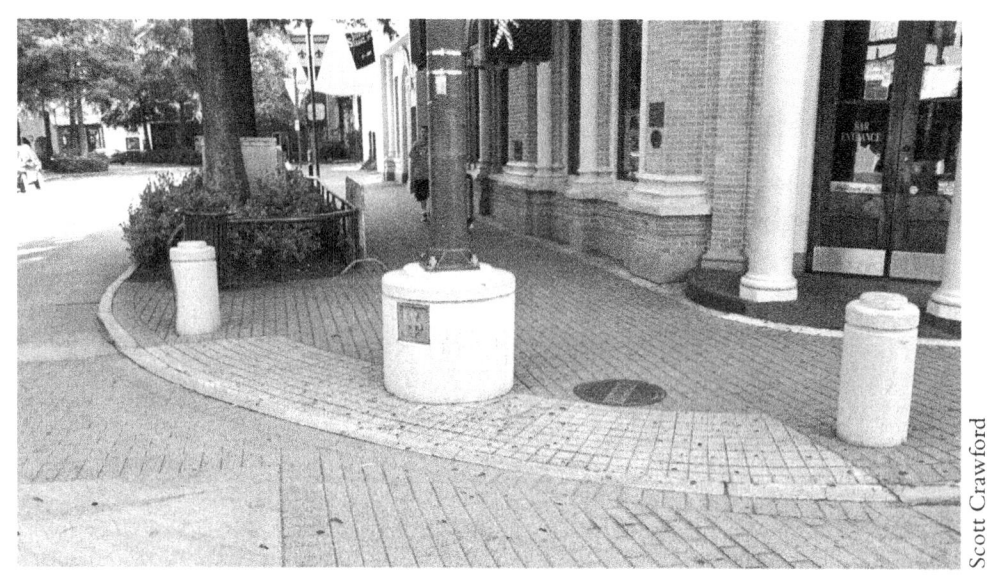

FIGURE **5.10**
Without a noticeable slope, materials intended to provide warning of a transition may not be tactilely discernible to visually impaired travelers.

The following questions can be used to guide identification of problems related to transitions:

- Are important transitions identifiable (such as from sidewalk to street or from countertop to stovetop)?
- Are there too many transitions that are insignificant, creating an overload of information?
- Are the transitions clear?

VIGNETTE STUDIES: APPLYING THEMES

The following vignettes are examples of applying the four themes to analyze problems and generate solutions.

Vignette 1: Missing Contrast and Transition Cues on Sidewalks

A gentleman working at a university in Atlanta traveled on foot from the bus stop to his office. As he followed the shoreline of the path (the boundary where the sidewalk meets the grass) along his route with his cane, sidewalks branched

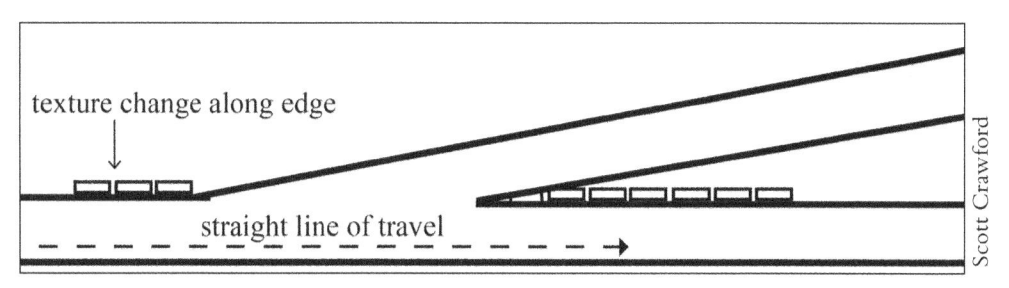

FIGURE 5.11
Transition Cue on Sidewalk
Bricks across the inside shoreline of the sidewalk provide texture to indicate branching pathway.

off from the main pathway at very slight, undetectable angles. This made distinguishing between the straight line of travel and the branching sidewalks difficult. The university installed bricks along the inside angle and in front of where the sidewalk branched off to provide a change in texture along the shoreline (see Figure 5.11). When the man reached the end of the bricks, he knew a path was branching off and he needed to leave the shoreline to maintain a straight line of travel to his office building.

Table 5.1 shows an analysis of the situation presented in the vignette according to the four themes and how this analysis generated the solution.

TABLE 5.1 Analysis of Vignette 1

Theme	Analysis	Solution
Consistency	No detectable difference between main and branching walkways.	Install brick indicators consistently at branching sidewalk junctions.
Contrast	Slight angle of sidewalk junctions does not provide enough contrast to signal change in direction.	Ends of brick indicators signal the locations of branching sidewalks.
Texture	No detectable difference in surface texture of main and branching walkways.	Brick indicators add texture along interior edge.
Transition	Change in sidewalk direction is too slight to be detected.	Ends of brick indicators signal the locations of branching sidewalks.

TABLE 5.2 — Analysis of Vignette 2

Theme	Analysis	Solution
Consistency	Grass ground surface is consistent throughout area—no detectable difference to indicate pathways.	Use logs to indicate routes of travel.
Contrast	Brown logs have little contrast with grass.	Paint logs white to increase visual contrast.
Texture	No variation in texture of grass.	None provided.
Transition	No detectable pathways.	Arrange logs to indicate paths of travel among buildings and pond.

Vignette 2: Missing Consistency and Contrast for Path of Travel

A woman with low vision who resides on a large piece of property in rural Georgia needed to be able to travel across grass fields between areas on the property. Her husband placed logs along the routes of travel through the grass, but these were still difficult to see because their brown color did not provide enough contrast against the grass. He then painted the logs white. The contrast between the white log and the green grass made it easy for her to navigate visually from her house to the barn, workshop, and pond. Table 5.2 shows the analysis of the environmental issues in this vignette.

Vignette 3: Missing Texture and Pathways

At a factory, lines taped and painted on the floor designated established pathways where products and equipment were not allowed. Other areas outside of the pathways contained hazardous overhangs and equipment. To provide a line that could be felt by employees with visual impairments, the lines were redone with a paint that included a nonskid compound (in this case, sand). The lines were painted slightly wider (6 inches) than the original lines (3 inches) to ensure that they were discernible. Table 5.3 shows the analysis of the environmental issues in this vignette.

Vignette 4: Missing Hazard Warning and Temporary Use

A committee chose a hotel for a conference without first visiting the hotel. The hotel had a lodge design that created architectural hazards for someone

TABLE 5.3 Analysis of Vignette 3

Theme	Analysis	Solution
Consistency	System of lines consistently indicates safe areas and pathways.	None needed.
Contrast	Lines on floor rely on visual contrast.	Increase width to enhance visibility of the line.
Texture	Lines lack texture detectable with a cane or under foot.	Add textural component (sand) to lines to aid in detection.
Transition	Transitions to and from safe areas are consistently indicated by lines.	None needed.

with a visual impairment. The steep, sloping ceilings could be hazards for head clearance if an individual with a visual impairment walked close to the wall, as he or she would when trailing the wall with a cane or fingertips. There were also large potted trees in the middle of the open areas and the wide hallways. When the hazards were discovered, there was little time to correct the situation. The existing potted plants were moved to specific areas along the walls where there was limited head clearance to block the hazardous areas (see Figure 5.12). The new location of the plants created tactile and visual contrast cues and a physical barrier to help people avoid the hazard. Conference participants were informed of the situation and where the environmental cues were placed. Table 5.4 shows the analysis of this environment.

SUMMARY

A wealth of environmental adaptation and modification resources are available with (1) tips for specific types of disabilities and age-related changes in vision, hearing, and mobility in home, community, and work environments; (2) information on technology and assistive devices; (3) guidance for understanding and navigating the ADA legislation and guidelines; and (4) information on principles for accessible design and construction. These can be found in the Resources section at the end of this book.

When older adults have low vision, environmental modifications and adaptations enable them to be as independent as possible in their pursuit of daily living skills, work, or recreational activities. Some of the adaptations made by older adults with low vision are intuitive and do not require a great

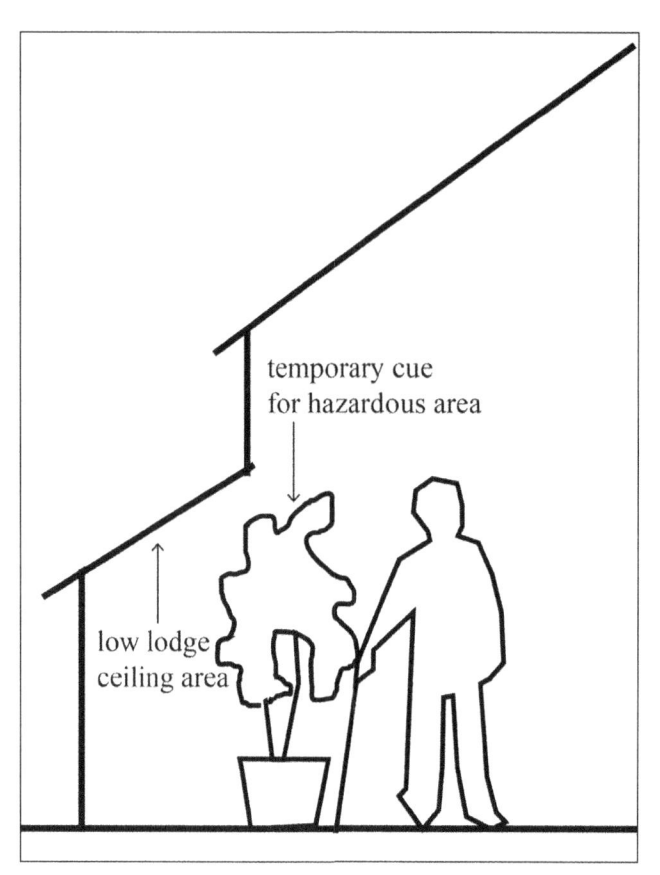

FIGURE **5.12**

Low Ceiling Hazard

Plants are a temporary fix for the low ceiling hazard.

TABLE 5.4 Analysis of Vignette 4

Theme	Analysis	Solution
Consistency	Area lacks consistent cues or warnings for locations of hazards.	Use potted plants to consistently indicate hazards.
Contrast	Lacking cues for hazard areas.	Location of potted plants to indicate a change in environmental conditions.
Texture	Lacking textural cues for hazard areas.	Use potted plants to indicate the transition between safe and hazardous areas.
Transition	Lacking cues for change in ceiling line and head clearance.	Use potted plants to indicate the transition between safe and hazardous areas.

deal of thought. However, creativity and problem solving on the part of professionals, family members, and the individuals themselves may be required when an obvious fix is not apparent. By applying the four themes for problem analysis and solution generation discussed in this chapter, effective solutions can be readily developed to meet the challenges faced by older individuals with low vision to accomplish tasks and pursue independence.

LEARNING ACTIVITIES

1. Review one of the resources for environmental adaptations and modifications found in the Resources section at the end of this book and apply the information to an elderly relative's home.
2. Analyze your workplace in regards to ADAAG compliance. Identify areas of concern and possible solutions.
3. Develop a vignette similar to the four mentioned earlier in the chapter and explore plausible solutions for consistency, contrast, texture, and transition.

References

Barlow, J. M., Bentzen, B. L., & Franck, L. (2010). Environmental accessibility for students with vision loss. In W. R. Wiener, R. L. Welsh, & B. B. Blasch (Eds.), *Foundations of orientation and mobility: Vol. I. History and theory* (3rd ed., pp. 324–384). New York: AFB Press.

Bradtmiller, B., & Annis, J. (1997). *Anthropometry for persons with disabilities: Needs for the 21st century* (Contract no. QA96001001). Washington, DC: U.S. Access Board. Retrieved from http://www.access-board.gov/research/completed-research/anthropometry-for-persons-with-disabilities-needs-for-the-21st-century

Griffin-Shirley, N., & Welsh, R. L. (2010). Teaching orientation and mobility to older adults. In W. R. Wiener, R. L. Welsh, & B. B. Blasch (Eds.), *Foundations of orientation and mobility: Vol. II. Instructional strategies and practical applications* (3rd ed., pp. 286–308). New York: AFB Press.

Guilford, J. P. (1967). *The nature of human intelligence.* New York: McGraw-Hill.

Michalko, M. (2001). *Cracking creativity: The secrets of creative genius.* New York: Ten Speed Press.

National Association of Home Builders. (n.d.). *Certified Aging-In-Place Specialist (CAPS).* Washington, DC: Author. Retrieved from http://www.nahb.org/en/learn/designations/certified-aging-in-place-specialist.aspx

Public Rights-of-Way Access Advisory Committee. (2007). *Accessible public rights-of-way planning and design for alterations* (Special Report). Retrieved from http://www.access-board.gov/guidelines-and-standards/streets-sidewalks/public-rights-of-way/guidance-and-research/accessible-public-rights-of-way-planning-and-design-for-alterations

Robinson, K. (2011). *Out of our minds: Learning to be creative*. West Sussex, UK: Capstone Publishing.

Sanford, J. A., Story, M. F., & Jones, M. L. (1997). An analysis of the effects of ramp slope on people with mobility impairments [Electronic version]. *Assistive Technology, 9*(1), 22–33. Retrieved from http://www.homemods.org/resources/ramp/index.html

U.S. Access Board. (2002). *ADA Accessibility Guidelines (ADAAG)*. Washington, DC: Author. Retrieved from https://www.access-board.gov/guidelines-and-standards/buildings-and-sites/about-the-ada-standards/background/adaag

U.S. Access Board. (2003). *ADAAG requirements for detectable warnings*. Washington, DC: Author. Accessed June 30, 2013, from http://c.ymcdn.com/sites/www.apbp.org/resource/resmgr/dpfa/adaag_requirements_for_detec.pdf

U.S. Access Board. (2014). *Detectable warnings update*. Washington, DC: Author. Accessed May 9, 2015, from https://www.access-board.gov/guidelines-and-standards/streets-sidewalks/public-rights-of-way/guidance-and-research/detectable-warnings-update

U.S. Access Board. (n.d.). *Outdoor developed areas regulatory negotiation committee members*. Washington, DC: Author. Accessed May 9, 2015, from http://www.access-board.gov/guidelines-and-standards/recreation-facilities/outdoor-developed-areas/background/regulatory-negotiation-committee-members

U.S. Department of Justice. (2010a). *2010 ADA standards for accessible design*. Washington, DC: Author. Accessed May 9, 2015, from http://www.ada.gov/regs2010/2010ADAStandards/2010ADAstandards.htm

U.S. Department of Justice. (2010b). *Guidance on the 2010 ADA standards for accessible design*. Washington, DC: Author. Retrieved from http://www.ada.gov/regs2010/2010ADAStandards/Guidance2010ADAstandards.htm

U.S. Equal Employment Opportunity Commission. (2008). *ADA Amendments Act of 2008*. Washington, DC: Author. Accessed May 9, 2015, from http://www.eeoc.gov/laws/statutes/adaaa.cfm

CHAPTER 6

Importance of Exercise for Orientation and Mobility for Older Adults with Visual Impairments

Laura Bozeman and Huan Zhang

With age, exercise and fitness for both the mind and body remain important to good health. This chapter presents four types of exercise suggested by the National Institute on Aging. Fall prevention is discussed and integrated into orientation and mobility (O&M) instruction, and resources and strategies for O&M professionals are provided.

EXERCISE AND HEALTH

Many adults lead a sedentary lifestyle; over 50 percent of adults do not exercise regularly (Haskell et al., 2007). According to the U.S. Department of Health and Human Services (2000), the statistics are even more discouraging for individuals with disabilities. Of the 54 million Americans with disabilities, less than half engage in regular, purposeful exercise. Furthermore, in older individuals with visual impairments, there are greater incidences of obesity, depression, and comorbid conditions than in the sighted population (Campbell, Crews, Moriarty, Zack, & Blackman, 1999; Crews & Campbell, 2001). Numerous research studies note a multitude of benefits from exercise, ranging from maintaining physical health to psychological well-being (Corn, Bina, & Sacks, 2008; Farrenkopf & McGregor, 2000).

The many benefits of exercise include overall fitness and improved health in general (Miszko, Ramsey, & Blasch, 2004). Ponchillia, Strause, and Ponchillia (2002) also noted how exercise promotes a level of flexibility that is important for the completion of daily activities. Increased strength and stamina are useful in emergencies and support independence. Integrated with these physical benefits are clear cognitive benefits from improved vascular performance, memory, and environmental awareness (Uemura et al., 2012). Exercise clearly improves strength, flexibility, and balance, which are known to help prevent falls (Griffin-Shirley & Welsh, 2010; Mancinelli, Mandich, & Utzman, 2011; Miszko et al., 2004). Medical conditions that are more common in the older adult, such as arthritis, diabetes, and hypertension, are better managed with consistent and appropriate exercise.

For older adults with visual impairments, safe and independent O&M is a key component of everyday life. Walking to the bus stop, to public transportation, and to nearby shops requires increased awareness, stability, and balance. In an emergency, an older adult may need to move quickly to avoid danger, requiring quick cognitive responses as well as strength and endurance (Uemura et al., 2012). Yet, when vision loss occurs, older adults may discontinue exercise programs or become more sedentary due to lack of transportation, depression, or the inability to travel independently. Excess pounds can put stress on hips and knees and can slow or halt O&M instruction. The ensuing lack of movement can make it easier to become overweight, creating a cycle that is difficult to break. Lack of exercise puts the older adult at risk for falls and deteriorating health that could lead to a cycle of decline (Johnson, 2005). While it is important to maintain an awareness of the many benefits of exercise, the O&M specialist will want to be aware of these and other possible barriers to consistent exercise, such as lack of accessibility and availability (Capella-McDonnall, 2007; Jones & Nies, 1996; Lieberman, Ponchillia, & Ponchillia, 2013), and plan instruction accordingly.

Aside from lack of accessibility and availability, there may be additional barriers to exercise. Research has shown that there is little encouragement or expectation for older adults with visual impairment to engage in fitness (Capella-McDonnall, 2007; Rimmer, Rubin, & Braddock, 2000). The staff at organized exercise facilities may not know how to accommodate and adapt exercises for participants with visual impairments. Health issues can also be a barrier to participating in exercise. Pain can act as an impediment, such as when an older adult with arthritis experiences pain with movement. Any physical condition that impacts stamina can also be seen as a barrier to fitness. Resistance may also come from the older adult who does not have the confidence or knowledge to participate in exercise. Even walking may seem unattainable if the older adult has not yet had O&M instruction, especially if the vision loss is recent.

EXERCISE OPTIONS

One of the most accessible and available opportunities for exercise is walking. Walking can improve cardiovascular function, stamina, and muscle tone and requires little specialized equipment. For the older adult with visual impairment, O&M instruction can promote and maintain safe and active walking for exercise. Another good option that is easy on the joints is water aerobics, although access to a pool may be a hindering factor for some. Another option is tai chi, a safe, easy, and fun way to increase stamina, promote balance, and increase independence (Miszko et al., 2004).

The baby boomer generation is quite active and is remaining active as they age (Wellner, 1998). With this level of activity, a range of fitness options are available to them. The National Institute on Aging (2011) recommends exercises for older adults that target four areas important to overall health: balance, endurance, strength, and flexibility.

Balance

Balance exercises are some of the most important types of exercises for seniors. As the age of the older adult increases, the risk of falls and resulting injuries increases (Griffin-Shirley & Welsh, 2010). A fear of falling can deter the older adult with visual impairment from physical activity and have a negative impact on fitness. A combination of medical assessment, environmental modifications, and exercise can improve balance and help prevent falls (Riddering, 2008; Steinman, Nguyen, Pynoos, & Leland, 2011). Activities such as walking, tai chi, water aerobics, and yoga all help strengthen muscles and improve balance (McGonigal, 2009; Riddering, 2008). If walking is not possible (due to health concerns) or transportation to organized fitness classes or a pool is a challenge, the older adult with visual impairment can use exercise machines or do chair exercises from their home (Lieberman et al., 2013). Leisure programs are available from health care programs and living options for adults 55 and over that include fitness alternatives geared to the abilities of the older adult. Most forms of purposeful movement contribute positively to improved balance.

Wallmann, Gillis, Alpert, and Miller (2009) studied the effect of a jazz dance class on the static balance abilities of women ages 54–88. The class met one time per week for 15 weeks. Results demonstrated significant improvement in static balance as measured by the Balance Master Sensory Organization Test, which evaluates a person's use of sensory systems that contribute to postural control (Wallmann et al., 2009).

Good balance is important in many areas of O&M as well as activities of daily living. Examples are negotiating stairs and activities that involve making a transition from one position to another, such as moving from sitting to standing. Gathering items to prepare a meal, collecting laundry, and basic household chores all require balance for safety.

Endurance

Endurance exercises are activities that are performed for at least 30 minutes. The purpose of endurance exercises is to build energy and stamina to stay in good shape. Walking, jogging, swimming, biking, and even vacuuming are all good examples of endurance activities for the active adult (National Institute on Aging, 2011). Tai chi is another good option for most older adults since it is a low-impact exercise that promotes flexibility, balance, and endurance. For the adult who prefers or requires a lower activity level, endurance can be addressed by using a treadmill or elliptical machine, performing chair exercises, or walking indoors (Lieberman et al., 2013).

For O&M, endurance is important for route completion and overall stamina. Endurance is a key factor in emergency situations, such as when needing to take an alternate, perhaps longer, route to avoid a dangerous situation, or when negotiating stairs in an evacuation.

Strength

Strength exercises are activities that strengthen muscles and increase metabolism. Strength exercises help keep weight and blood sugar in check. Classes that use stretch bands to develop muscle strength can be easily adjusted to the individual's ability. Stretch bands or light weights that can tone and strengthen can also be used at home. Mall walking, jogging, and swimming are all good exercises for strength (National Institute on Aging, 2011). Dance classes or dancing for entertainment (square-dancing, ballroom dancing, dancing at a party) are all enjoyable ways to keep fit and not only develop strength, but improve endurance and keep weight under control.

Flexibility

Flexibility exercises are based on stretching. Stretching can be practiced from standing and sitting positions. Yoga and tai chi are examples of activities that place an emphasis on flexibility exercises.

Moving more freely (flexibility) makes it easier to reach upper cabinets, or reach down to put on a shoe (National Institute on Aging, 2011). Locating dropped objects (retrieving a dropped cane, for instance) involves stretching and flexibility. Reduced flexibility can alter the older adult's gait and posture and can result in a tendency to veer to one side or the other, which can lead to problems with orientation.

BENEFITS OF TAI CHI

There are many activities that combine the four exercise types mentioned earlier. Tai chi is one of the best options, especially for older adults. It is described here in some detail as an example of how exercise can be beneficial for older adults in general and specifically for improving O&M skills.

Tai chi is a holistic approach that stresses physical and psychological balance through low-impact, low-intensity, controlled movements. Tai chi motions are easy on the joints and focus on developing physical conditioning and mental peace through balance, relaxation, and increased circulation (see Figure 6.1)

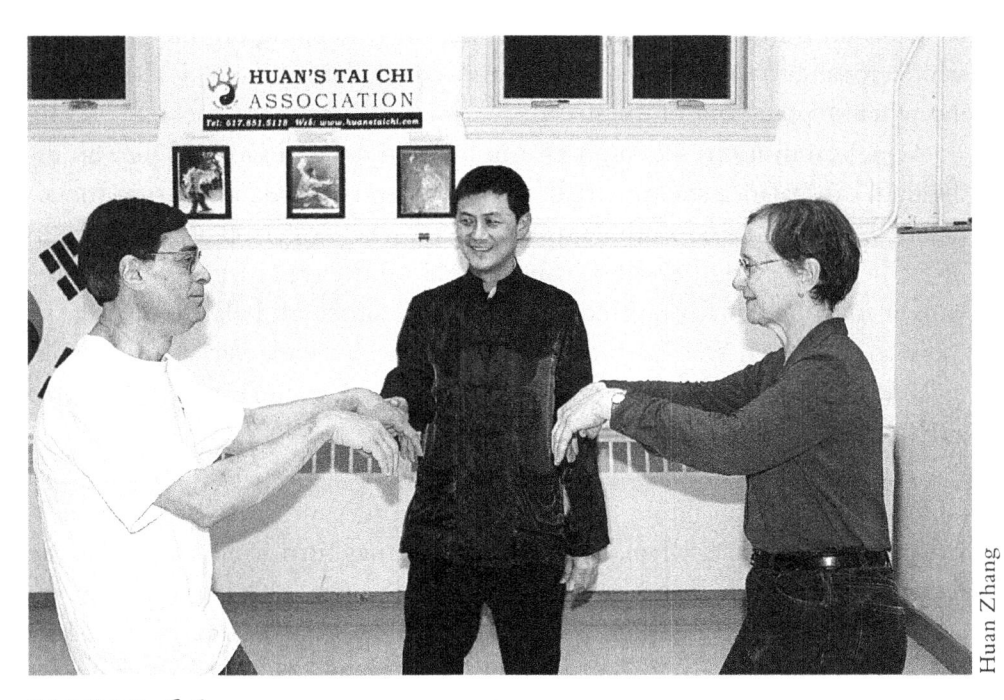

FIGURE **6.1**
Huan Zhang demonstrates tai chi's opening form to two older adults during a lecture at his studio.

(Miszko et al., 2004). Tai chi opens the joints and increases strength and endurance. Tai chi has been termed "meditation in motion" for its smooth and elongated movements and is currently one of the most popular exercises for seniors of all ages in China and many other parts of the world (Jacoby & Youngson, 2005).

The movements of tai chi have been practiced by Chinese people for many years. As with many fitness programs, the benefits of tai chi are both physical and psychological. Physical benefits include strength, flexibility, and balance. Psychologically, the exercises reduce stress and promote feelings of well-being (Miszko et al., 2004).

Many tai chi principles to help keep the body balanced, energetic, strong, and flexible are also important to O&M, as well as in preventing falls. These include central equilibrium, weight transitions, coordination, and concentration (Yang, 1934/2005).

Central equilibrium is the foundation of tai chi and refers to balanced movement; it is the key to both initiating movement and to subsequent movements. For a person with a visual impairment, this equilibrium is critical to the safe negotiation of a task. For example, when crossing a street, central equilibrium is important at the beginning when stepping off into the street, while crossing to maintain purposeful movement, and at the end of the crossing when stepping out of the street.

Weight transitions are important in both tai chi and O&M. Once an individual can balance standing still, the next step is to balance during movement. Weight transition problems can occur when a person attempts to lift his or her first leg while still bearing weight on the other leg. In tai chi, the weight must be equally shifted, maintaining consistent balance during the transfer. In O&M, weight shifting plays a part in a wide variety of actions, including stepping off of and onto curbs, negotiating stairways, and starting and stopping momentum.

Tai chi places a lot of emphasis on coordination. Tai chi uses the waist to control coordination rather than trying to coordinate each body part individually. For example, when walking, a person may turn at the waist to swing the right arm forward and step out with the left leg. This process is an example of coordination. Coordination between the right arm and left leg balances the movements and the body. In O&M, coordination is the basis for many techniques, including the three-point touch technique and the contralateral (opposite side) components of keeping the cane in step with the feet in the two-point touch technique (Jacobson, 2013).

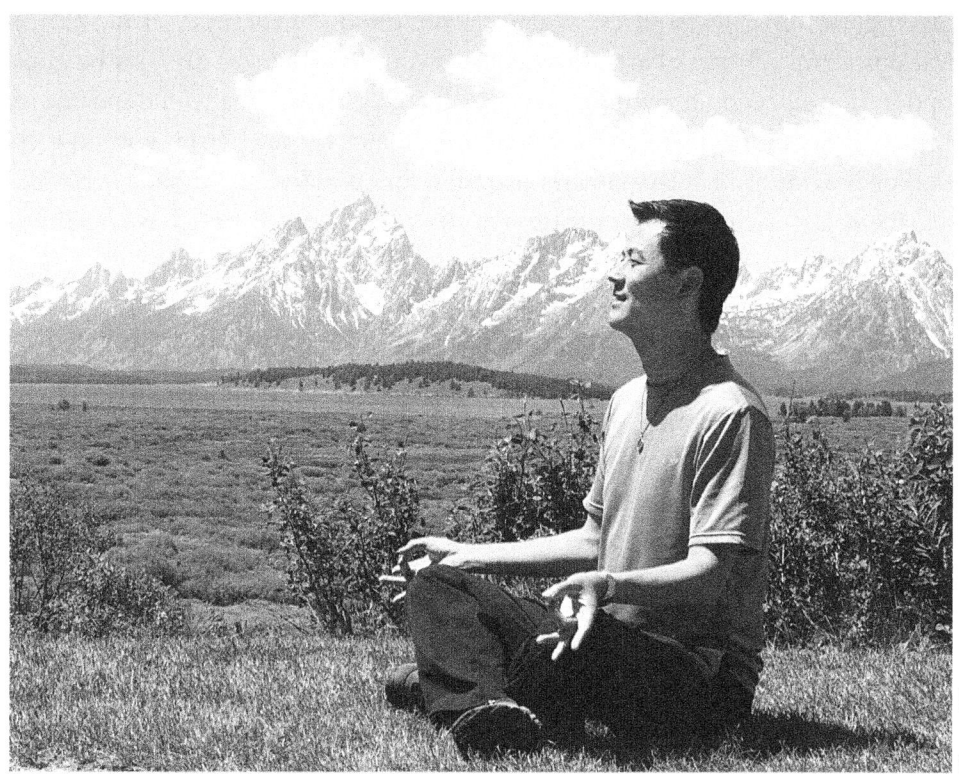

FIGURE **6.2**
Huan Zhang demonstrates a mind relaxation exercise in front of the Grand Teton Mountains.

Tai chi is also a lesson in concentration (see Figure 6.2). One mind cannot be used for two things simultaneously, or the quality of one or the other will suffer. In O&M, as well as tai chi, multitasking can cause problems. For example, if a person is walking and listening to his or her phone, he or she might not concentrate on the surrounding environment or pay attention to the road conditions. He or she may be more likely to run into something, trip, or fall. Tai chi emphasizes performing tasks one at a time (Fu, 1963/2006).

ADDITIONAL FITNESS OPTIONS

There are many options for the older adult to engage in exercise and fitness. Organized sports are good options for active older adults, especially sports specifically designed for individuals with visual impairments, such as goalball and beep baseball. In these games, if a player is sighted or has remaining vision, playing customarily requires wearing a blindfold. (Lieberman et al., 2013). Various forms of martial arts, such as tae kwon do or karate, can also be good options for older adults with visual impairments. Adaptations would include an instructor standing close and modeling movements for the person with low vision or providing a hands-on demonstration for an individual with no vision.

Exercise classes are good opportunities for fitness as well as socialization. Jazzercize, yoga, Zumba, and water aerobics are examples. An adapted demonstration of the moves may be necessary initially, and then the older adult with visual impairment can follow the music or guidance provided by the instructor.

Some fitness options require little or no specialized equipment and can be done in various environments or at home. Walking can be done at any intensity that works best for the older adult and can occur outdoors or in a mall or other indoor environment. Chair exercises also make use of equipment readily available to the older adult and can be done at home. Exercise machines, such as a treadmill, elliptical, or stationary bike, require the apparatus but can be done at any time and at the intensity desired by the individual. If obtaining the equipment is a barrier, community organizations are often able to help. The Lions Club has various locations throughout the country and often provides support to individuals with vision and/or hearing impairments.

HELPING CLIENTS BEGIN AN EXERCISE PROGRAM

Since O&M is a critical part of life for the older adult with visual impairment, fitness can be the key to continued independence and participation for that person. Often, O&M is the method for accessing exercise classes or establishing a fitness routine that involves walking. The routes used during training may be incorporated into the routine of the older client.

When working with older adult clients to begin an exercise program, it is important to obtain permission from the client's physician for any physical activity that constitutes a significant change from the person's typical routine. The O&M instructor may advocate for low-impact exercise such as walking or tai chi. It is always a good idea to suggest that older adults increase physical activity slowly and incrementally. Depending on the type of exercise, a client may be advised to increase intensity or duration a little bit on a daily or weekly basis.

If the client is exercising in a facility or taking a class, the O&M specialist should meet with the personal trainer or exercise program instructor to discuss how instruction and guidance can be modified to include verbal cues, how to model positions, and how physical prompts can be used effectively. (See Lieberman et al., 2013, for detailed information about how various physical activities can be adapted for people with visual impairments and ways of providing instruction when an individual cannot see the instructor.) For this reason, the topic of advocacy is important when beginning a fitness class. The older adult with visual impairment needs to know the accommodations he or she needs to participate in the activity. Often, the fitness class instructor will not be sure how to accommodate a person with vision loss. Making sure the older adult is prepared and knowledgeable about available accommodation options will help both the older adult and the instructor. Sidebar 6.1 presents a number of strategies that O&M specialists can use to help motivate older adults to exercise.

SIDEBAR 6.1

Strategies to Facilitate Exercise for Older Adults with Vision Loss

O&M specialists can use the following strategies to motivate older clients with vision loss to participate in physical fitness activities.

- Have older adults try new recreational activities with a friend or family member.
- Plan transportation and practice routes to and within a client's fitness facility to help the client move around independently.
- Make sure any educational materials offered by a client's fitness facility are provided to the client in an accessible form to ensure he or she is well informed.
- Suggest older adults maintain exercise journals to track the effects of exercise and its impact on O&M.
- Experiment with low vision devices to determine which devices work best for specific activities.
- Role play advocating for accommodations or interacting with exercise instructors when necessary.

Source: Griffin-Shirley, N., & Welsh, R. L. (2010). Teaching orientation and mobility to older adults. In W. R. Wiener, R. L. Welsh, & B. B. Blasch (Eds.), *Foundations of orientation and mobility: Vol. II. Instructional strategies and practical applications* (3rd ed., pp. 286–311). New York: AFB Press.

FALL PREVENTION

Falls are the primary cause of accidental death in people over 65 years of age (Fuller, 2000). In that age group, 30 to 40 percent of people will fall; the percentage is increased for those with visual impairments (Slay, 2002).

A combination of medical assessment, exercise and physical activity, and environmental modifications is the best approach to successful fall prevention (LaGrow, Robertson, Campbell, Clarke, & Kerse, 2006; Steinman et al., 2011). A cross-disciplinary approach to fall prevention includes physical therapists, occupational therapists, physicians, and social workers in addition to the vision professionals on the team (Gleeson, Sherrington, & Keay, 2014). This level of collaboration allows thorough assessment of the individual's medical status (including the side effects of prescription drugs), physical capabilities, visual abilities, and an environmental evaluation to eliminate trip hazards and barriers in the home. (Sidebar 6.2 provides suggestions for eliminating hazards in the home that can cause falls.) As noted previously, the improved strength, flexibility, and balance that can be derived from exercise and fitness can help to prevent falls.

Mancinelli et al. (2011) note that O&M specialists are examples of professionals who can assess functional visual abilities as well as the environment for hazards that can affect safety. The O&M specialist, in collaboration with other related service professionals, can determine the preliminary risk for falls.

SUMMARY

Exercise is critical to maintain health, movement, and balance. Exercise for older adults is important for these reasons and to maintain quality of life. Older adults with visual impairment should make use of all strategies that fit their individual lifestyles to keep active, fit, and mobile. Fitness is an integral part of O&M and a foundation for safe and independent travel. The rehabilitation team can support fitness as well by integrating therapy or treatment into the routine of the older adult with visual impairment. Occupational and physical therapists can support fitness with exercises that mimic the older adult's movement goals and activities. O&M specialists can consult with older adults, their family members, and other professionals to assist adults with vision loss to engage once again or begin a new exercise program that is enjoyable, easy to do, maintains movement and balance, and meets their needs for a healthy quality of life.

SIDEBAR 6.2

Safety in the Home: How to Eliminate Hazards and Be Safe

Implementing the following suggestions can help older people with visual impairments prevent falls and improve safety in their homes.

- Eliminate small throw rugs; they can cause tripping.
- Make sure the bath mat has a nonskid backing.
- Keep electrical cords as close to the baseboards as possible and out of walkways.
- Keep floor lamps and small items, such as low tables, magazine racks, and plants, out of walkways.
- Clean up spills immediately. If you forget about a spill, you might slip on it.
- Close cabinet, closet, and cupboard doors and drawers completely to avoid accidentally running into them.
- Pick up shoes, clothing, books, and other items that can cause you to trip. Put away an object when you are through using it—for safety and to help in locating it again.
- Do not store objects in high places that require the use of a step stool for retrieval.
- Arrange furniture so that there is a clear path for walking and keep clutter out of walkways.
- Avoid using furniture on wheels.
- Use clap-on/clap-off lights to adjust lighting without getting up from a chair or bed.

Source: Adapted from VisionAware. (n.d.). *Preventing falls*. New York: American Foundation for the Blind. Retrieved from http://www.visionaware.org/info/everyday-living/home-modification-/safety-in-the-home/preventing-falls/1234; VisionAware. (n.d.). *Safety in the home*. New York: American Foundation for the Blind. Retrieved from http://www.visionaware.org/info/everyday-living/home-modification-/safety-in-the-home/123

LEARNING ACTIVITIES

1. Participate in a local tai chi class. Note how this form of exercise benefits you as well as older people in the class.

2. Visit a senior center and interview the activities director about the exercise programs for older adults offered there. Observe one of the classes and note if accommodations would be needed for an older adult with visual impairment to participate.

3. Interview an older adult with vision loss regarding his or her exercise routine.

References

Campbell, V. A., Crews, J. E., Moriarty, D. G., Zack, M. M., & Blackman, D. K. (1999). Surveillance for sensory impairment, activity limitation, and health-related quality of life among older adults: United States, 1993–1997. *CDC Morbidity & Mortality Weekly Report, 48*(S S08), 131–156.

Capella-McDonnall, M. (2007). The need for health promotion for adults who are visually impaired. *Journal of Visual Impairment & Blindness, 101*(3), 133–145.

Corn, A. L., Bina, M. J., & Sacks, S. Z. (2008). *Looking good: A curriculum on physical appearance and personal presentation for adolescents and young adults with visual impairments.* Austin, TX: Pro-Ed.

Crews, J. E., & Campbell, V. A. (2001). Health conditions, activity limitations, and participation restrictions among older people with visual impairments. *Journal of Visual Impairment & Blindness, 95*(8), 453–467.

Farrenkopf, C., & McGregor, D. (2000). Physical education and health. In A. J. Koenig & M. C. Holbrook (Eds.), *Foundations of education: Vol. II. Instructional strategies for teaching children and youths with visual impairments* (2nd ed., pp. 437–463). New York: AFB Press.

Fu, Z. (2006). *Mastering Yang style taijiquan* (L. Swaim, Trans.). Berkeley, CA: Blue Snake Books. (Original work published 1963).

Fuller, G. F. (2000). Falls in the elderly. *American Family Physician, 61*(7), 2159–2168.

Gleeson, M., Sherrington, C., & Keay, L. (2014). Exercise and physical training improve physical function in older adults with visual impairments but their effect on falls is unclear: A systematic review. *Journal of Physiotherapy, 60*(3), 130–135.

Griffin-Shirley, N., & Welsh, R. L. (2010). Teaching orientation and mobility to older adults. In W. R. Wiener, R. L. Welsh, & B. B. Blasch (Eds.), *Foundations of orientation and mobility: Vol. II. Instructional strategies and practical applications* (3rd ed., pp. 286–311). New York: AFB Press.

Haskell, W. L., Lee, I. M., Pate, R. R., Powell, K. E., Blair, S. N., Franklin, B. A., . . . Bauman, A. (2007). Physical activity and public health:

Updated recommendation for adults from the American College of Sports Medicine and the American Heart Association. *Medicine & Science in Sports & Exercise, 39*(8), 1423–1434.

Jacobson, W. H. (2013). *The art and science of teaching orientation and mobility to persons with visual impairments* (2nd ed.). New York: AFB Press.

Jacoby, D. B., & Youngson, R. M. (2005). *Encyclopedia of family health: Vol. 3* (3rd ed.). Tarrytown, NY: Marshall Cavendish.

Johnson, M. L. (Ed.). (2005). *The Cambridge handbook of age and ageing.* Cambridge, UK: Cambridge University Press.

Jones, M., & Nies, M. A. (1996). The relationship of perceived benefits of and barriers to reported exercise in older African American women. *Public Health Nursing, 13*(2), 151–158.

LaGrow, S. J., Robertson, M. C., Campbell, A. J., Clarke, G. A., & Kerse, N. M. (2006). Reducing hazard related falls in people 75 years and older with significant visual impairment: How did a successful program work? *Injury Prevention, 12*(5), 296–301.

Lieberman, L. J., Ponchillia, P. E., & Ponchillia, S. V. (2013). *Physical education and sports for people with visual impairments and deafblindness: Foundations of instruction.* New York: AFB Press.

Mancinelli, C. A., Mandich, M., & Utzman, R. R. (2011). Physical therapy approach to falls in adults with visual impairment. *Insight: Research and Practice in Visual Impairment and Blindness, 4*(3), 124–132.

McGonigal, K. (2009). *Yoga for pain relief: Simple practices to calm your mind and heal your chronic pain.* Oakland, CA: New Harbinger Publications.

Miszko, T. A., Ramsey, V. K., & Blasch, B. B. (2004). Tai chi for people with visual impairments: A pilot study. *Journal of Visual Impairment & Blindness, 98*(1), 5–13.

National Institute on Aging. (2011). *Exercise & physical activity: Your everyday guide from the National Institute on Aging.* Bethesda, MD: U.S. Department of Health and Human Services, National Institutes of Health. Retrieved from http://www.nia.nih.gov/health/publication/exercise-physical-activity

Ponchillia, P. E., Strause, B., & Ponchillia, S. V. (2002). Athletes with visual impairments: Attributes and sports participation. *Journal of Visual Impairment & Blindness, 96*(4), 267–272.

Riddering, A. T. (2008). Keeping older adults with vision loss safe: Chronic conditions and comorbidities that influence functional mobility. *Journal of Visual Impairment & Blindness, 102*(10), 616–620.

Rimmer, J. H., Rubin, S. S., & Braddock, D. (2000). Barriers to exercise in African American women with physical disabilities. *Archives of Physical Medicine and Rehabilitation, 81*(2), 182–188.

Slay, D. H. (2002). Home-based environmental lighting assessments for people who are visually impaired: Developing techniques and tools. *Journal of Visual Impairment & Blindness, 96*(2), 109.

Steinman, B. A., Nguyen, A. Q. D., Pynoos, J., & Leland, N. E. (2011). Falls-prevention interventions for persons who are blind or visually impaired. *Insight: Research and Practice in Visual Impairment and Blindness, 4*(2), 83–91. Retrieved from http://www2.allenpress.com/pdf/aerj-04-02-83-91.pdf

Uemura, K., Doi, T., Shimada, H., Makizako, H., Yoshida, D., Tsutsumimoto, K., . . . Suzuki, T. (2012). Effects of exercise intervention on vascular risk factors in older adults with mild cognitive impairment: A randomized controlled trial. *Dementia and Geriatric Cognitive Disorders EXTRA, 2*(1), 445–455.

U.S. Department of Health and Human Services. (2000). *Healthy people 2010: Understanding and improving health* (2nd ed.). Washington, DC: U.S. Government Printing Office.

VisionAware. (n.d.). *Preventing falls.* New York: American Foundation for the Blind. Retrieved from http://www.visionaware.org/info/everyday-living/home-modification-/safety-in-the-home/preventing-falls/1234

VisionAware. (n.d.). *Safety in the home.* New York: American Foundation for the Blind. Retrieved from http://www.visionaware.org/info/everyday-living/home-modification-/safety-in-the-home/123

Wallmann, H. W., Gillis, C. B., Alpert, P. T., & Miller, S. K. (2009). The effect of a senior jazz dance class on static balance in healthy women over 50 years of age: A pilot study. *Biological Research for Nursing, 10*(3), 257–266.

Wellner, A. S. (1998). Getting old and staying fit. *American Demographics, 20*(3), 24–27.

Yang, C. (2005). *The essence and applications of taijiquan* (L. Swaim, Trans.). Berkeley, CA: Blue Snake Books. (Original work published 1934)

CHAPTER 7

Daily Living Skills and Orientation and Mobility
Merging Skills to Enhance Life Satisfaction

Gretchen Good and Laura Bozeman

Orientation and mobility (O&M), or the skills required to be oriented and move around safely in various environments, including in one's own home, are central to virtually every daily activity (Ponchillia & Ponchillia, 1996). O&M skills are important both as isolated techniques and when used in combination with other adaptive techniques, as integrated strategies for independent living (Guth, Rieser, & Ashmead, 2010).

For older people, independent mobility is central to maintaining many important life roles. O&M specialists benefit from understanding how O&M and other daily living skills are linked. Health, memory, stamina, and expectations can all have an impact on how older individuals retain life roles and cope with vision loss. The purpose of this chapter is to suggest ways in which daily living and O&M skills can be merged, with the cooperation and coordination of various professionals, for older adults with visual impairments. The result should be enhanced life satisfaction, which is the ultimate goal of rehabilitation. Specific topics are highlighted that have been linked to life satisfaction for older adults with visual impairments, including low vision rehabilitation, recreation, driving, and activity and independence in general. Community living facilities, safety, and emergency preparedness are discussed. The chapter ends with a more in-depth discussion of the concept of life satisfaction and a review of the principles of adult learning as they apply to older adults with visual impairments.

O&M AND OTHER AREAS OF INDEPENDENT LIVING

O&M involves skills that are also necessary for independent living and for daily activities. For example, in order to read the mail, a person with a visual impairment needs to first safely move to retrieve the mail using cane techniques, trailing techniques, environmental information, and orientation principles and then perhaps use adapted lighting, magnification, and eccentric viewing skills to access the mail. Confident and safe movement is necessary for many leisure, recreation, and home-management skills.

Twelve domains of independent living for older people (Good, 2005) have been established and are listed in Table 7.1. Many activities of daily living (ADL) also require skills in O&M. ADLs have been defined as tasks completed throughout the course of the day and can include both basic activities of daily living (BADL), such as personal-care tasks like toileting and dressing, and more complex instrumental activities of daily living (IADL), such as shopping, cooking, and community activities (Good, 2005).

TABLE 7.1 Independent Living Domains Requiring O&M Skills

Domain of Independent Living	Example of Task Requiring Both O&M and Daily Living Skills
Basic activities of daily living (BADL)	Transferring from chair to car, couch, or wheelchair
Personal management	Managing medications (such as picking up prescriptions from pharmacy)
Caring for others	Looking after grandchildren
Home management	Sweeping floors
Kitchen management	Putting away groceries
Outdoor home maintenance	Raking leaves
Clothing care	Hanging laundry
Communication	Accessing mail
Recreation outdoor	Walking or jogging
Recreation indoor	Dancing
Community participation	Going to movies, plays, concerts
Managing money	Using a money machine for banking

Source: Good, G. A. (2005). *Ageing and vision impairment: Activity, independence and life satisfaction.* Unpublished doctoral thesis, Massey University, Palmerston North, New Zealand. Retrieved from http://muir.massey.ac.nz/bitstream/10179/1542/1/02_whole.pdf

A number of professionals may work with older people who are visually impaired, and their specializations often overlap. Each team member can benefit from understanding his or her role as well as the roles of other specialists in assisting older people with visual impairments to improve their satisfaction with daily living in each of the domains listed in Table 7.1. Sidebar 7.1 lists the scope of practice of these professionals. Generally, orientation and mobility specialists teach concepts and travel skills to people with visual impairments and provide strategies for individuals to know where they are in space and to travel safely, efficiently, and as independently as possible. Vision rehabilitation therapists teach people with impaired vision strategies in the areas of communication systems, personal management, home management, leisure and recreation, psychosocial aspects of blindness and vision loss, medical management, and basic O&M skills, including human guide and safety techniques. The scope of practice of low vision therapists involves identification of visual impairments and use of functional vision evaluation instruments to assess vision and teach the use of visual perceptual and visual-motor skills. Professional teams may also include a social worker, recreation specialist, occupational/physical therapist, and sensory integration specialist.

Frequently, professionals dually certified in both O&M and vision rehabilitation therapy can provide a rehabilitation program to individuals needing extensive O&M and instruction in adaptive daily living skills. If an older adult's O&M needs are primarily related to movement within familiar indoor environments, the O&M instruction may be delivered by a vision rehabilitation therapist. In addition, a number of professionals other than low vision therapists—including vision rehabilitation therapists and orientation and mobility specialists—can also provide training in the use of low vision devices.

MOST IMPORTANT ACTIVITY AND INDEPENDENCE AREAS

O&M specialists and other professionals can utilize research to help them create meaningful rehabilitation plans for their older clients with visual impairments. In a study involving 560 older adults (Good, 2005), visual impairment had a negative impact on the frequency of activity for older adults in the areas of outdoor and indoor work, leisure, and mobility. Interestingly, activities in the domestic domain (such as cooking and cleaning) did not decrease in frequency. Specific tasks in which older people with visual impairments were much less active when compared to those with sight included driving, reading,

SIDEBAR 7.1

Professionals Who Teach O&M and/or Daily Living Skills

These descriptions of professionals who work with older adults as part of the vision rehabilitation team refer to their role in teaching O&M and daily living skills. For more general information about the responsibilities of some of these professionals, see Sidebar 1.3 in Chapter 1.

O&M SPECIALISTS

O&M specialists teach people with visual impairments a sequential process to utilize their senses, determine their position, and negotiate safe movement (Academy for Certification of Vision Rehabilitation and Education Professionals, 2014). These professionals also teach concepts and spatial awareness.

VISION REHABILITATION THERAPISTS

Vision rehabilitation therapists teach people with visual impairments strategies to support communication, personal management, home management, leisure and recreation, psychosocial aspects of blindness and vision loss, medical management, and basic O&M skills, including human guide and techniques for increased safety. They can teach the use of compensatory skills and assistive technology and work with clients to enhance vocational opportunities, independent living, and educational development (Academy for Certification of Vision Rehabilitation and Education Professionals, 2015).

LOW VISION THERAPISTS

Low vision therapists use functional vision evaluation instruments to assess effective use of vision and teach visual perceptual and visual-motor skills as well as the use of low vision devices. The low vision therapist can evaluate work history, educational performance, quality of life, and performance of daily living skills (Academy for Certification of Vision Rehabilitation and Education Professionals, 2015).

OCCUPATIONAL THERAPISTS

Occupational therapists work to reduce disability and promote independence and participation in meaningful activities. Occupational therapists can be part of a coordinated team working with visually impaired adults to enable them to participate in their communities, age in place, gain independence in living, and be productive. Occupational therapists use therapeutic strategies to teach activities of daily living that promote a return to work.

> Occupational therapists can also be involved in driving assessment and rehabilitation (Warren & Nobles, 2011).
>
> **PHYSICAL THERAPISTS**
>
> Physical therapists help maximize range of motion and balance as well as using exercise to restore function and "develop, maintain and restore maximum movement and functional ability throughout the lifespan" (World Confederation for Physical Therapy, 2014).
>
> Physical therapists can also be part of a rehabilitation team working with older people with visual impairments. Physical therapists "help people maximize their quality of life . . . , which encompasses physical, psychological, emotional and social wellbeing" (World Confederation for Physical Therapy, 2014). They may be involved in health promotion, providing treatment and interventions, and modify environments.

gardening, going for car rides, household maintenance, using a typewriter or computer, and work (paid or volunteer) (Good, 2005, 2008).

In 2008, Good examined areas of independent living that created dissatisfaction and difficulty for older people with visual impairments. Areas shown to be most difficult were outdoor work and community activities. Older people with and without vision loss were dissatisfied with their independence in community involvement and recreation, both areas that require strong O&M and daily living skills (Good, 2008). Independent living domains in which those with visual impairments were significantly less independent than their sighted peers were found to be handling money, community involvement, and caring for others.

Acquiring a vision loss often means older people must give up activities that are important to them. Good (2005) demonstrated that the relinquished activities most closely related to a lower quality of life for those with visual impairments included dancing, sexual activity, shopping, visual entertainment (such as watching television), and going out at night.

This information could be useful in designing rehabilitation programs for older clients and helping people retain their ability to engage in important activities. O&M specialists will want to address areas that research suggests are most important to their older clients early in rehabilitation programs, working with daily living specialists (such as occupational and physical therapists or vision rehabilitation therapists) to help clients achieve independence, interdependence, and satisfaction in their daily lives. These areas include the following:

- tasks that seem to affect older adults who are visually impaired, such as reading and driving, as opposed to skills that are affected mostly by age, such as outdoor home maintenance, so that clients can gain skills to function similarly to their sighted peers
- tasks that cause the most dissatisfaction for those with impaired vision, such as recreation
- tasks that older adults with visual impairments rate as the most difficult, such as going out to movies, plays, and concerts
- tasks that when relinquished are most closely related to lower life satisfaction, such as dancing and shopping

Among these tasks, research indicates that when recreation and driving are relinquished, they result in the most diminished life satisfaction (Good, 2005), so those areas will be discussed in more detail later in this chapter.

It is also important to prioritize activities of daily living and O&M skills necessary for survival and safety, such as medication management, kitchen management, safe travel in familiar environments, emergency preparedness, and backup plans, discussed later in this chapter.

Rehabilitation professionals need to understand the unique needs and desires of each individual client in order to deliver appropriate O&M, ADL, low vision, or other rehabilitation services. Working from standardized checklists may not always reveal a client's frustrations, strengths, weaknesses, or desires for activity and independence after significant loss of vision, as shown in the following example:

> Mr. Cooper, a 72-year-old man, has macular degeneration that has affected his ability to read standard print. He is an avid sportsman and spectator. Even though reading print may appear to be his most significant and most recent activity limitation, when asked to prioritize his rehabilitation needs, he reported that he really missed watching baseball from the stands. He stated that his wife has always dealt with the daily mail in their home and although he enjoys reading, he likes the Talking Books he receives. Therefore, finding low vision distance devices to enable him to continue to watch baseball is his most important goal.

LOW VISION SERVICES, DEVICES, AND TECHNOLOGY

There is good evidence that low vision services (assessment, prescription of low vision devices, and training in their use) are linked to improved life satisfaction and have a large, positive effect on clinical reading ability (reducing the size of print that can be read and increasing reading speed) (Binns et al., 2009). Low vision service has been described as "a rehabilitative or habilitative package which provides a range of services for people with low vision to enable them to make the best use of their eyesight to achieve maximum potential" (Palmer, 2005, p. 4). In addition, low vision devices are valued and used by people with visual impairments (Binns et al., 2009). O&M specialists, vision rehabilitation therapists, low vision therapists, and other team members can all provide functional training in using low vision devices.

For older adults, low vision services are thought to be important to enable them to continue in valued activities using their remaining vision. Although older adults are likely to have experienced vision loss, they may still have usable vision and are often inclined to use visual, rather than nonvisual, adaptations. Both nonvisual skills as well as techniques to better use remaining vision should be incorporated into the rehabilitation service plan. There is evidence that when low vision services are integrated into a comprehensive rehabilitation service plan that includes both O&M and instruction in daily living skills, instead of being delivered separately, the result is better outcomes and improved perceptions of quality of life (LaGrow, 2004).

Low vision devices and technology are useful to older people in many activities of daily living. There are five types of low vision devices (Minto & Butt, 2004).

1. convex lens devices such as spectacle, handheld, and stand-mounted magnifiers (including illuminated models)
2. telescopic systems, either spectacle-mounted or handheld
3. nonoptical (adaptive) devices such as large print, lighting, reading stands, marking devices, and talking clocks, timers, and scales
4. tinted lenses and filters, including antireflective lenses
5. electronic reading systems such as desktop and portable video magnifiers, optical print scanners, computers with large-print programs, and computers equipped with voice commands to access the programs

In a study conducted in the United Kingdom (Palmer, 2005), participants noted their functional use of low vision devices for the following activities, in descending order of frequency:

1. reading the paper
2. reading instructions
3. reading letters
4. reading TV guide
5. reading bills, receipts, hymns
6. reading bank statements
7. watching TV
8. seeing controls on oven
9. reading food packets and cans
10. reading medicine labels
11. doing crossword puzzles
12. identifying bus numbers
13. sorting money
14. reading recipes
15. knitting
16. playing lawn bowls (similar to bocce or other lawn games)

The factors that promoted use of low vision devices included ease of use, possibility of quick success, how much they aided independence, availability of training and support, availability of options, and whether the user had a positive attitude (Palmer, 2005).

Low vision services have been linked to moderate improvements in life satisfaction and quality of life. O&M and other specialists can work together in providing these services to help older adults with visual impairments retain meaningful activities of daily living and maintain life satisfaction.

THE IMPORTANCE OF RECREATION

Recreation has proved to be an area of vital importance to older adults with visual impairments (Good, 2005; Good & LaGrow, 2000). In Good's (2005) study, recreation was the activity most highly correlated with positive life satisfaction in older people with impaired vision. Recreation was also the area in which the most dissatisfaction was reported. Older adults with recent visual impairment reported that the onset of vision loss made them feel robbed of their opportunities for leisure and recreation activities during retirement, when their formal work responsibilities had diminished or ended.

Given the importance of recreation that was found in this research, it needs to be made a priority in rehabilitation programs for older people with visual impairments. Recreation is also important to people who are newly blind as a way to escape their fears and losses. If an individual cannot escape into a book or a movie or go for a walk, he or she may constantly be reminded of the vision loss. In addition, the peer support that can be experienced during recreational activities with others can smooth the process of rehabilitation. This is why it is important to be able to modify and adapt leisure and recreational activities to include individuals who are blind or visually impaired. Recreational activities can also help reinforce and provide opportunities to practice skills learned in O&M and ADL programs. People with impaired vision have interests as varied as those of anyone else. Professionals can help individuals learn strategies to adapt valued activities so they can be enjoyed despite vision loss (see Sidebar 7.2). (For more information about how to adapt recreational activities, see Lieberman, Ponchillia, & Ponchillia, 2013; Orr & Rogers, 2006).

Audio or e-books, talking watches and clocks, sunglasses, large-print books, playing cards, and puzzles are just some of the resources that can be introduced to older people to enable them to participate in valued activities. Sidebar 7.3 lists a number of recreational activities and sports that can be adapted for older adults who are visually impaired. Active participation can begin to make a difference in the lives of those with visual impairments. O&M professionals can enhance this participation and the life satisfaction of their clients by introducing recreation-oriented resources within O&M programs, as in the following example.

> Mrs. Taylor has vision loss as a result of diabetic retinopathy. She lives in a retirement village and has previously enjoyed regular card games and walks with her neighbors. An O&M specialist, in collaboration with a vision rehabilitation therapist, can work with Mrs. Taylor to adapt to large-print playing cards and to introduce the cards to her card group. Together, the professionals can also teach Mrs. Taylor to confidently use the guide technique with a friend and to reduce glare with sunshields. They can also recommend routes to Mrs. Taylor and her walking companions. Eventually, long cane instruction can be a part of Mrs. Taylor's plan.

SIDEBAR 7.2

Tips for Including Older Adults with Vision Loss in Recreational Activities

The following techniques can help older adults participate in their favorite recreational activities:

- Help clients recognize their interests, skills, and talents and make modifications so they can be included in activities.
- Have older adults make use of other senses.
- Use positioning to make best use of remaining vision.
- Have the individual substitute touch techniques for visual observation.
- Narrate and describe what is happening in the environment and/or what the support person is doing.
- Introduce low vision devices and modifications.
- Eliminate barriers and negative attitudes by helping the client realize that many activities are possible with little or no adaptations. Often just showing the client how things can be done is the key. For peers and service providers who do not personally live with impairments, contact with people with disabilities can reduce prejudice, stigma, and stereotypes.

DRIVING AND OLDER ADULTS WITH VISION LOSS

Those who have had to stop driving report lower levels of active recreation, lessened participation in life roles, and a decrease in overall life satisfaction (Liddle, Gustafsson, Bartlett, & McKenna, 2012). Older adults often experience vision loss gradually, over a long period of time (Ryan, Anas, Beamer, & Bajorek, 2003). An important threshold occurs when it is no longer safe for an individual to continue driving. This can be a heartbreaking dilemma for older people and their families. O&M specialists may be ideally placed to help individuals and families make such an important determination and to find dignified alternatives to independent driving. It could be useful to have access to other professional advice (from a driving specialist, for example) during this time.

The privilege of driving is just that—a privilege—although many people view driving as more of a right. Driving represents independence and con-

SIDEBAR 7.3

Recreational Activities and Sports for Older Adults with Visual Impairments

ACTIVITIES THAT ARE EASILY ADAPTABLE TO NONVISUAL TECHNIQUES

The following are some of the recreational activities that can be adapted relatively easily for people with visual impairments:

- amateur radio
- board games
- card games
- clay, pottery, and dough
- paper craft
- leather craft
- weaving
- yarn crafts
- dance and drama
- photography
- music
- woodworking
- writing
- taped correspondence
- sewing
- genealogy
- beadwork
- travel
- cooking
- computers

SPORTS ACTIVITIES OFTEN ORGANIZED FOR VISUALLY IMPAIRED AND MIXED GROUPS

The following are some group activities that can be easily adapted to include people with visual impairments:

- sailing
- tandem bicycling
- hiking
- skiing
- swimming
- fencing
- lawn bowling
- golf
- fishing
- goalball
- athletics
- ten-pin bowling
- water skiing
- wrestling
- cricket
- hockey

trol over a person's life, and so it is often not relinquished lightly. In many areas there are not many options for travel for older adults who cannot drive independently. Bus routes and stops are not always convenient or safe. Inclement weather makes walking to and waiting for buses uncomfortable and unsafe for some older people. Taxis are not always available and are often unaffordable. Managing groceries and packages while using public transportation is not always feasible. Hiring drivers, soliciting rides, and using specialized transport for people with disabilities may be difficult for older individuals to accept, especially if they have travelled independently all of their lives. The spontaneity offered by independent travel is difficult to replicate by other means. And if an individual is reliant on public transportation, it can limit where he or she can live. In our society, automobiles are symbols of socioeconomic standing, independence, and responsibility; driving is also an expected social norm. A great deal of work must be done with clients who can no longer drive to develop strategies for using optical devices (where appropriate) and arranging transportation, and for coping with the frustrations of being unable to drive.

Restrictions on Driving with Impaired Vision

There is little unanimity throughout the world regarding vision standards for driving; often, whether or not someone can see well enough to drive safely has to be considered on an individual basis. Vision specialists are required to make life-altering decisions about an individual's ability to drive while balancing the ethics of respecting a patient's confidence and simultaneously attempting to protect the public good. The O&M specialist may play a valuable role in helping clients assess their ability to perform the visual skills needed for safe driving. Sidebar 7.4 summarizes some of the barriers to safe driving related to vision issues in older adults and the conditions that may cause them.

Loss in the visual field occurs with aging, according to Turano et al. (2004). Although monocular vision (vision loss in one eye) creates challenges to safe driving and some studies report up to seven times more accidents in those with monocular impairments (Politzer, n.d.), those with "some field loss or monocular vision seem to be able to drive safely, compensating by increasing their head movements and using other clues for distance judgment." Many transportation authorities do not cite monocular vision as a reason for disqualification, as long as one eye has a full visual field (Politzer, n.d). Politzer (n.d.) recommends the use of optical aids such as wide mirrors and both passenger and driver-side mirrors for those driving with monocular vision.

A driver aware of his or her functional vision may be able to compensate well enough and drive safely. On the other hand, the contribution of poor vision to motor vehicle accidents is likely to be underestimated. It is difficult to establish that poor vision has contributed to an accident, but studies by the American Optometric Association (Shipp et al., 2000) have shown that mandatory vision testing for re-licensure can have benefits in the form of improved safety records.

It is interesting to note that diplopia (double vision) is noted as a driving hazard only if the onset is recent. Individuals are advised to seek advice if

SIDEBAR 7.4

Vision-Related Barriers to Safe Driving in Older Adults

Visual conditions that may serve as a barrier to safe driving in older adults include the following:

- Decreasing visual acuity
- Binocular field defects
- Dyplopia (double vision)
- Reduced night vision and resistance to glare
- Reduced light and dark adaptation
- Impairment of depth perception
- Reduced visual processing speed

These barriers can be caused by conditions such as the following:

- High myopia
- Cataracts
- Glaucoma
- Keratoconus
- Diabetic retinopathy
- Macular degeneration

Source: Huss, C. P. (2012). *Prerequisites for rehab specialists involved in the low vision driver education training and assessment process.* Bioptic Driving Network.

---

they develop this condition, but may be able to eventually drive again safely (NZ Transport Agency, 2009).

Impairments of color vision alone do not have a correlation with accidents and generally require no driving restrictions (NZ Transport Agency, 2009). Impairment of color vision that prevents a driver from perceiving the color of traffic lights can easily be compensated for by noting the position of traffic lights, as they have generally been standardized. Note, however, that horizontal traffic lights and arrows require the individual to memorize the configuration of the traffic lights.

Because the ability to adapt to changes in dark and light conditions decreases with age, someone with poor adaptation skills will likely have difficulty when suddenly entering a long and dark road tunnel, a parking garage, or when getting stranded in traffic after dark. Yet there are no available statistics that back a claim that this is a significant contribution to accidents. It is likely that people with adaptation difficulties self-regulate their driving to avoid such situations.

Requirements for driving with impaired vision vary from state to state in the United States (Huss & Corn, 2004; Lee & Ponchillia, 2010; Marta & Geruschat, 2004). Conditions can be listed on drivers' licenses, including the following:

- must wear prescribed lenses
- occlusion must be worn
- external mirrors must be fitted on both sides of the car (some states and countries do not require two side-mounted mirrors)
- daytime driving only
- regular medical assessment required
- types of roads can be restricted (for instance, no highway driving)

In over 40 U.S. states, the use of a bioptic telescope system can enable a person to obtain a license, if the spectacle-mounted monocular helps the person achieve 20/40 acuity and have at least 20/120 or 20/100 acuity through the carrier lens. Not much research is available about safety and bioptic driving, but it appears that safety records are comparable to drivers who are not visually impaired (Owsley, 2012). Other research shows conflicting conclusions about the safety of bioptic driving. Concerns include how well bioptic drivers manage curves, turns, required weaving maneuvers, and rapid stops (Luo & Peli, 2011).

Historically, some ophthalmologists have been opposed to the use of bioptic lenses for driving (Fonda, 1983), and an individual can only use bioptic telescopes to drive legally in 43 U.S. states as well as Holland and Quebec (Bowers & Krader, 2013; Luo & Peli, 2011, Owsley, 2012). Some think it is possible that these lenses make it legal for a person to drive but not necessarily safely (Luo & Peli, 2011). Those who have been prescribed a bioptic telescope system and who anticipate being able to use them for driving will want to seek the expertise of driving instructors, O&M specialists, low vision specialists, and certified vision rehabilitation therapists to undergo an appropriate training program to ensure safe use of bioptics for driving. Individuals may be required to complete an approved training program with a set number of training and practice hours before a license is approved and issued. It is important to search each state's requirements before suggesting bioptic driving to a client. (For more information on driving with a bioptic telescope system, see Huss & Corn, 2004; Lee & Ponchillia, 2010.)

Older drivers are thought to make more mistakes due to inadequate surveillance, misjudgment of the length of a gap between vehicles, and misjudgment of another vehicle's speed (Cicchino & McCartt, 2015). Additionally, older drivers in general can be more fragile and more likely to be injured or killed in an accident (Donorfio, D'Ambrosio, Coughlin, & Mohyde, 2009).

The following are some suggestions for drivers with visual impairments:

- Wear your eyeglasses when driving.
- Be aware of night vision reduction and problems with glare as you get older and consult an ophthalmologist if you note problems, as it may indicate early development of cataracts.
- If you lose the vision in one eye, allow yourself adjustment time to learn compensatory judgment skills.
- Consider installing extra rear vision mirrors.

There are many issues concerning driving and visual impairment. The people who make decisions about fitness to drive and those who have the power to revoke licenses, as well as drivers and their families who question a driver's ability to be safe on the road, have many factors to consider. Balancing individual freedom, patient confidentiality, and the public good is not an easy task. Often, licensing regulations related to vision are liberal, which leaves room for potentially fatal mistakes, but also allows for flexibility and individualized decisions.

Psychological Impact of Not Driving

Being an individual who no longer drives in an automobile-oriented society is a "transportation disability" (Corn & Sacks, 1994, p. 67). The psychological impact of being an adult who no longer drives has not been explored in great depth. Even general literature on disability omits transportation as an issue. The effects of not being able to drive include great inconvenience and a variety of challenges that can pose logistic, psychological, practical, and financial barriers to freedom and independence. The following are some common challenges and considerations faced by people who no longer drive:

- preplanning means of transportation (inability to be spontaneous)
- walking in dangerous areas alone
- requesting rides from others
- ensuring security while in transit alone
- paying for transportation
- relying on others' time and schedules
- accepting rides
- carrying objects throughout the day
- explaining to others why one cannot drive
- being unable to go places not served by mass transit
- waiting for others or for public transportation
- being unable to attend important functions

These challenges, and the frustrations they can cause, should not be minimized. People who no longer drive often must make major adjustments to their lifestyles. They lose choice in living options and must have cash available to pay for transport services. Professionals sometimes fail to consider the impact not driving can have on an individual's sense of true independence and control over his or her life. The grief of facing relinquishment of driving rights can be substantial. These needs must be addressed as part of any rehabilitation process.

O&M and other vision specialists, as well as occupational and physical therapists and driving rehabilitation specialists can assist in the evaluation of driving skills of older adults through clinical and functional assessments. Professionals can communicate assessment results and recommendations to clients and can provide remedial driving courses, adaptive driving instruction and retraining, and rehabilitation and vehicle modification. Huss (2012) provides a list of 13 prerequisites for rehabilitation specialists to assist in the low vision driver education training and assessment process (see Sidebar 7.5).

Professionals can educate the public so groups may offer transportation to all who might need it, not just targeting older adults for rides to church functions, community, and recreation events. For example, community groups that rely on volunteers may be able to recruit from a much wider pool of skilled volunteers if they were to offer those with impaired vision transportation or payment for taxis, to enable qualified volunteers to work in schools, museums and hospitals. People with disabilities can be given instruction in

SIDEBAR 7.5

Prerequisites for Rehabilitation Specialists Involved in the Low Vision Driver Education Training and Assessment Process

1. Review your state's rules and regulations regarding vision standards for driving.

2. Know your opposition (if transportation officials or medical professionals do not want to allow an individual with low vision to drive) and attempt to resolve differences on issues without litigation or legislation.

3. Review those college notes regarding the anatomy, physiology and pathology of the eye.

4. Be aware that individuals with the same visual disorder will function and interpret the world (including dynamic driving environment[s]) around them differently.

5. Access and preview audio-visual driver education training materials, such as the I.P.D.E. (identify, predict, decide, and execute) process, defensive driving skills, and safe space-cushion driving principles.

6. Learn how to operate audio-visual equipment correctly and independently.

7. Observe firsthand the differences and similarities of the driving performance(s) of sighted versus low vision driver education students and clients.

8. Obtain formalized driver evaluation training that incorporates standardized methods for observing, evaluating, and rating the performance of drivers.

9. Become familiar with and able to recognize pre-driver readiness and awareness abilities of your assigned clients (for example, remembering and following instructions, traveling designated routes, detecting and reacting to objects or conditions, or analysing traffic-controlled intersections).

10. Enhance your knowledge of various visual characteristics—such as visual acuity, contrast sensitivity, useful field of view, and visual field—and their relevance to the driving task.

(continued)

> **SIDEBAR 7.5** (*continued*)
>
> 11. Review your state's driver's manual (especially regarding pavement markings, road signs, and road laws).
> 12. Become knowledgeable regarding various types, styles, and powers of bioptic telescopic lens systems (including correct use and areas of concern of each system).
> 13. Become a good listener.
>
> ---
>
> *Source:* Reprinted with permission from Huss, C. P. (2012). *Prerequisites for rehab specialists involved in the low vision driver education training and assessment process.* Bioptic Driving Network.

how to request and accept transportation. When an individual must stop driving, O&M specialists and other professionals can assist in finding alternative means to maintain important life roles and life satisfaction.

STRATEGIES FOR INDEPENDENCE IN COMMUNITY LIVING FACILITIES
The Need for Knowledge and Understanding

For older adults with visual impairments who live in communal settings such as independent or assisted living centers, it is important that those around them understand the functional implications of specific eye conditions. A caregiver should understand that someone with age-related macular degeneration and a central vision loss may be able to travel well yet may not be able to see details to read, sew, distinguish colors, or identify faces. Understanding specific eye conditions can explain puzzling behavior from a resident in a long-term care facility. For example, a caregiver may be frustrated when a resident cannot identify the caregiver's face (because of a loss of central vision), but can identify a coin rolling across the floor (using peripheral vision).

Residential facilities should ideally have staff members who understand the functional implications of cataracts, glaucoma, age-related macular degeneration, and diabetic retinopathy (see Chapter 2 for more information about specific conditions). In addition, staff members need to be aware of Charles Bonnet Syndrome, a neurological phenomenon affecting some older adults with visual impairments, described in Chapter 2. The functional implications of Charles Bonnet Syndrome include hallucinations and may last up to 12 to 18 months (Royal National Institute of Blind People, 2015). Staff members sometimes wrongly assume that older adults with this visual condition have dementia.

Undetected cataracts can result in problems with lighting and glare and the need for frequent changes of eyeglass prescriptions, which may not improve vision. The functional implications of glaucoma could include loss of peripheral vision, which can mean that an individual may have difficulty moving around and avoiding obstacles, yet be able to read or see a clock across the room. A white cane can be useful to someone in this situation but residential staff may not have an understanding of the cane or its use. Facility personnel should also understand the extreme frustration of fluctuating vision that is related to diabetic retinopathy.

There are higher rates of vision loss (3 to 15 times higher) for older adults who live in residential care facilities than those who live in the community. Estimates are that 33 percent of these older residents in residential care facilities could improve function through simple correction (lenses). Correcting poor vision for these older adults has been shown to reduce depression (Owsley et al., 2007).

Misunderstandings and miscommunication among staff, older residents, and family members can be alleviated if everyone gains an understanding of the implications of these eye conditions. Staff training needs to be well structured, give specific strategies and information, and provide basic information about working with older adults with visual impairments (see Sidebar 7.6). People working in residential care must understand that each person with vision loss will have unique needs. O&M professionals can be involved in providing education to staff about eye conditions, thus potentially improving the lives of those adults with vision loss.

Environmental Modification and Safety in Residential Care Facilities
Basic Environmental Modification

Safety is an important issue to address for those living in residential care facilities. A variety of hazards can be found in residential care facilities, particularly for people with visual impairments, such as area rugs, electrical cords, cluttered traffic areas, and shin bumpers (e.g., coffee tables), which can cause falls. Making facilities, programs, and activities safe as well as comfortable

> **SIDEBAR 7.6**
>
> ## Basic Skills for Residential Home and Assisted Living Staff When Working with Older People with Visual Impairments
>
> It is sometimes the role and responsibility of O&M specialists and other rehabilitation professionals to provide guidance to staff of facilities on working with older adults with visual impairments. The following are some basic suggestions that can be offered:
>
> - Introduce yourself to an adult with a visual impairment by name.
> - To offer assistance, touch your hand to the back of his or her hand.
> - Let the resident know when you are leaving the area.
> - Direct him or her to a comfortable waiting spot before you walk away; for example, ensure proper support is available.
> - Do not do a task for someone if the individual prefers to do it without assistance.
> - Describe the surroundings when appropriate.
> - Use a clock face analogy when describing the location of food on a plate.
> - Push chairs under the table when vacating them so that residents will not bump into them.
> - Keep doors entirely opened or closed to avoid accidental collisions.
> - Keep cupboard doors closed.
> - Use guide techniques.

and accessible for older people with visual impairments does not need to cost great amounts of time or money, however. The key is knowledge of the basics in using lighting, color, contrast, glare reduction, and furniture configuration and to develop awareness of hazards, hallways, stairs, and signs. Part of an O&M professional's role may be to assess safety and recommend changes to improve safety for those with vision loss in their own homes or in community living situations. (See Chapter 5 for additional discussion of assessing and modifying the environment to meet the needs of older people with visual impairments.)

Lighting. Floor and table lamps can be used to provide direct and overhead lighting. Use adjustable blinds and arrange chairs and tables near windows to make good use of natural light and enhance the visual functioning of those with low vision in residential settings (Duffy, 2002).

Glare. Glare can be reduced with the use of adjustable blinds and sheer or net curtain linings. Sunglasses and visors, worn inside, can make a dramatic difference in an individual's ability to navigate through and around sunny interior areas. Make sure that individuals do not have to view television or people in front of bright, glaring backgrounds such as bare windows.

Furniture Configuration. Furniture can be arranged into small groups to make conversation easier for those with hearing and vision difficulties. Good lighting can be provided in these furnished spaces to enhance conversation. Textured fabrics can help people identify which couch or chair they have found, and bright accessories, such as contrasting throw pillows and blankets, can assist people to find the particular seat they seek. It can be helpful to avoid the use of complex patterns on floor coverings and furniture.

Color and Contrast. Bright colors and contrast can be useful. Dark furniture against a white wall, use of contrasting placemats and plates, doorframes painted in contrast to the walls, contrasting doorknobs and switch plates, and brightly colored strips on stairs, steps, and ramps can all help make life easier for those with visual impairments who live in residential settings.

Hazard Indications. Hallways and stairs can be made safer with uniform lighting, grab bars, contrasting color on landings, and bright, secure mats to provide contrast at the tops and bottoms of stairways. Accessible signage should be large, tactile, positioned at eye level, and contrasting, printed in black text on a white or yellow background.

Fire Safety

Fire safety protocols in residential facilities must be reviewed frequently and escape plans must be practiced repeatedly. Practicing fire safety, rather than relying on improved fire-fighting technology, is the most effective means by which people who are blind or visually impaired can improve their chances of surviving a fire. O&M professionals can be involved in assisting in emergency safety planning in residential homes—as they do in schools—helping to identify safe routes, barriers, and backup plans. (General emergency preparedness is discussed later in this chapter.)

Some fire safety issues are unique to those with visual impairments. For example, high-decibel smoke alarms can interfere with auditory cues someone with vision loss needs for mobility. Many buildings are not equipped with useful signage for those with vision loss, putting them at increased risk for injury and disorientation. Large, open-air living spaces, such as are often found in community living facilities, can increase the spread of toxic gases and smoke. Newly developed directional audible signals may enhance safety. Directional sounders allow designers to create audible exit signs and map routes to the nearest exit using broadband, multifrequency sound. Guiding evacuees along an escape route, the alarms produce increasingly faster patterns of sound as a person gets closer to an exit (Boer & Withington, 2004).

To reduce the risks of depression and to improve life satisfaction for those with visual impairments who live in residential care, O&M and other specialists can work together to enhance environments and teach skills to individuals and staff that facilitate improved quality of life, inclusion, and safety.

EMERGENCY PREPAREDNESS: THE NEED FOR O&M AND DAILY LIVING SKILLS

"[The earthquake] made me feel terrible, useless is the word, useless, because if I had to run, I couldn't" (Margaret, 2011, older adult, survivor with visual impairment of New Zealand earthquake) (Good, Phibbs, Williamson, & Chambers, 2012).

Emergency preparedness has been linked with higher levels of life satisfaction (Gowan, Kirk, & Sloan, 2014). Recent natural disasters around the world have had many rehabilitation professionals thinking about the importance of being prepared to survive comfortably in the instance of an earthquake, flood, fire, power outage, loss of water service, and the like. Assisting older adults with visual impairments develop plans and strategies to cope in emergencies should become a part of all rehabilitation programs. O&M professionals may be ideally placed to assist individuals and communities with disaster preparation and response plans.

There is limited research on the experiences of people with vision loss in major disasters. However, people with disabilities are more likely to be poor and living in low-income neighborhoods—two factors that have been identified as risk factors for vulnerability to earthquakes (Chou et al., 2004). Living in a lower socioeconomic status, a person is likely to have fewer resources for coping in a disaster and fewer resources for recovering, and is more likely to experience stress and have a prolonged recovery (Wilkinson & Marmot, 2003).

Research in the area of emergency preparedness generally targets those who do not have disabilities. People with disabilities are likely to have greater health care needs, to live alone, and to be unable to respond quickly in an emergency (Chou et al., 2004).

Good, Phibbs, Williamson, and Chambers (2011) interviewed a group of adults with vision loss following the earthquake in Christchurch, New Zealand, in 2010. Those interviewed said they were reluctant to evacuate their homes because of concerns that emergency shelters would not be able to meet their needs. People within this group had a range of unmet health care needs after the disaster, as well as financial hardship, difficulties accessing health services, and difficulty obtaining medications. They also had concerns about orientation, mobility, housing, heat, electricity, water supplies, and transportation (Good et al., 2011; Good et al., 2012; Phibbs, Woodbury, Williamson, & Good, 2012).

Comorbidity factors that may contribute to blindness, such as diabetes and hypertension, are likely to put older adults who are blind at even greater risk during a disaster and throughout the recovery period. Themes that emerged from interviews with 12 mostly older earthquake survivors with visual impairments included communication and technology, support, O&M, and personal safety and health (Good et al., 2012; Phibbs et al., 2012).

Communication and Technology

Participants reported that the radio became a very important tool for communication. Those who could use an accessible cell phone, and those who did not have access to such a phone, reported that texting was, or could have been, an important medium for receiving information and maintaining contact with others. It seemed that GPS technology was of limited value in the wake of a disaster as GPS navigation tools were not up to date about routes that remained accessible.

Support

Participants made it clear that personal contact with friends, family, and even strangers was crucial to well-being. Little agency support was available in the days following the disastrous earthquake, so personal contact made all the difference.

Travel

Lack of standards for the erection of temporary building barriers, scaffolding, and security fences created difficulty in navigating neighborhoods. Participants had great difficulty getting out of their homes to pharmacies, friends, or service agencies. Dangerous obstacles created barriers to independent travel in areas affected by the earthquake as well as in the temporary service areas put up by local authorities. Participants reported great difficulty using canes and dog guides. Temporary roadways and bus routes disrupted individual routines, such as getting to appointments and to friends and family.

Personal Safety and Health Issues

Older people with vision loss who experienced the 2010 earthquake reported that they experienced an erosion of a sense of security and an increased sense of endangerment to their safety and health (Good et al., 2011). In the initial moments after the earthquake, there was the danger of stepping on broken dishes, glass, and fallen objects. Telephones and televisions did not work. Some reported that they did not know how safe their homes were or whether they should stay inside or venture outside, where they might encounter large crevasses, pools of water, and other hazards. In the days following the disaster, many reported difficulty with accessing medications if they required a complex regime of medications. Those who relied on oxygen had concerns about how they could evacuate. With the ongoing aftershocks, many reported a heightened sense of fear, panic, and an inability to sleep. Navigating one's own neighborhood was frightening and sometimes impossible.

The public was directed to service areas to obtain potable water and access portable toilets. Personal chemical toilet kits were made available, but these required the user to read the instructions for handling the chemicals and to carry the contents and dispose of it in large bins—very difficult to manage for a person who is blind.

Evacuation centers are not built to meet the needs of those with complex needs or disabilities. Evacuation centers can be cluttered and difficult to navigate. Centers are often located in large buildings with open gymnasium-type rooms for people to sleep in, providing few landmarks for travelers who are blind. These centers may or may not be suitable for dog guides, and often evacuees are required to fill in forms, read notices, and follow written instructions—all difficult or impossible when one is blind or visually impaired.

Professionals serving people with vision loss could work together with civil defense authorities to ensure that plans are made to help those who need assistance when emergencies occur. Professionals in the field of blindness and visual impairment could also work with individuals to have a plan in place if an emergency should occur. And those working in the field of aging and visual impairment could work with residential home staff to ensure that measures are in place to assist those who are blind or visually impaired in case of a large-scale emergency.

LIFE SATISFACTION, VISUAL IMPAIRMENT, AND ACTIVITIES OF DAILY LIVING

Life satisfaction "generally refers to a personal assessment of one's condition, compared to a reference standard, or to one's aspiration" (Garcia & McCarthy, 1995, p. 22). One perspective on aging is that the majority of older people age with some diminished functioning but little loss of satisfaction, happiness, independence, and meaningful activity. Classic researchers Carroll (1961) and Cummings and Henry (1961), for example, imply that older individuals can have improved satisfaction with their functioning because they have lowered expectations of themselves as they age. Current research also supports this view (Schnittker, 2007). Another perspective is that aging is characterized by profound and significant loss (Orr, 1991).

Research has demonstrated clear links between impaired vision and depression, communication breakdown, psychological dysfunction, decreased well-being and quality of life, lowered mood, and disrupted social relationships in those who are older (Belsky, 1999; Carabellese et al., 1993; Crews & Campbell, 2001; Dargent-Molina, Hays, & Breart, 1996; Heine & Browning, 2002; Horowitz, Leonard, & Reinhardt, 2000; Horowitz, Reinhardt, Boerner, & Travis, 2003; Stuen, 1999; Swagerty, 1995; Williams, Brody, Thomas, Kaplan, & Brown, 1998). But little has been done to investigate the links between visual impairment, activity and independence, and life satisfaction.

As noted earlier, Good (2005) investigated what matters most to older people in terms of daily functioning. Life satisfaction, satisfaction with independence, satisfaction with activity, satisfaction with social supports, as well as social comparisons of functioning were explored through 560 surveys and 60 interviews. Two groups participated: those with impaired vision and those with no impairment of vision. Those with visual impairments did report a lower level of life satisfaction overall. Visual impairment was found to be associated with lower levels of satisfaction with activity and independence in older people.

People are said to compare themselves with others in many ways to judge their own life situations, according to Leon Festinger (1954), who developed the social comparison theory. The theory basically states that there is a drive within individuals to gain accurate self-evaluations by comparing themselves to others. Overall, the difference in the proportions of those with impaired vision who, using social comparisons, compared themselves unfavorably to their peers was significantly higher than it was for those who were sighted. An exception was that at the oldest ages (85 and older), proportionally more sighted participants said that they functioned less actively and independently than their peers. The oldest participants with visual impairments did not report this perception as frequently.

Unexpectedly, the oldest age group with visual impairments reported a higher level of overall life satisfaction than did their sighted peers in the oldest age cohort as well as in comparison to younger cohorts with impaired vision. This improvement in life satisfaction in the oldest group of those with impaired vision has been linked to flexibility and cognitive adjustments in coping for those who have already experienced a great loss such as loss of vision. This may enhance coping skills and flexibility in comparison to sighted peers (Hamarat et al., 2002).

This study also included an exploration of factors that may contribute to life satisfaction for older people. Despite a moderate relationship between activity and independence and life satisfaction, activity and independence did not contribute significantly to overall life satisfaction. Significant predictors of life satisfaction included factors such as satisfaction with social support, and favorable social comparison of activity. Life satisfaction was also found to be positively correlated with the size of the individual's social support network. Having a greater number of health impairments was linked to lower life satisfaction, as was having relinquished a greater number of activities in the past five years. Overall life satisfaction was not found to be significantly linked to age, gender, marital status, income, or living situation (alone or with others) (Good, 2005).

When asked what contributed to and detracted from life satisfaction, a group of participants with impaired vision reported that their personal relationships and independence contributed to their life satisfaction with proportionally greater frequency than their sighted peers. Poor vision was mentioned as the primary detractor from quality of life by about 70 percent of those with vision loss who responded to the open-ended question. No other factor was mentioned as frequently.

Visual impairment clearly has a negative effect on life satisfaction. However, it has been determined that it does not appear to be limited activity and independence that create this lower level of life satisfaction. Still unknown is just which aspects of living with a visual impairment result in lower life satisfaction.

Favorable social comparisons of activity and independence were significantly correlated with life satisfaction in this study. Further, favorable social comparison of activity was found to be a significant independent contributor to life satisfaction, but only for those who had impaired vision. This is an important and unexpected finding, although it is logical. People with impaired vision are likely to experience compromised activity and independence. Although they may not be as active and independent as they once were, they may still be doing well in comparison to some peers because many older people are relinquishing activities for a variety of reasons as they age. Comparison to others has been demonstrated to be important in previous studies (Heidrich & Ryff, 1993; Ybema & Buunk, 1995). "Social comparison is receiving increasing recognition as an important strategy for adaptation in old age" (Frieswijk, Buunk, Steverink, & Slaets, 2004, p. 250). Results of the Good (2005) study discussed here, with favorable social comparison being one of the most notable contributors to life satisfaction for participants with impaired vision, are further validation for the need for subsequent investigation.

By comparing themselves with age peers in similar situations, older people can make an adjusted assessment that allows them to reinterpret their present lives in a positive manner. In this way, they can preserve their life satisfaction despite age-related loss. Social comparison has been shown to be more predictive of life satisfaction than factors such as aspiration level or comparison with one's prior situation (Emmons & Diener, 1985). O&M specialists and other rehabilitation professionals, if aware of the importance of social comparisons, can help clients see their levels of activity and independence in the context of their peers and to make comparisons that enhance life satisfaction.

THEORIES OF LEARNING AND METHODS FOR TEACHING OLDER ADULTS WITH VISION LOSS

Since research has shown that older adults with visual impairments find it important to compare their level of activity and independence favorably to peers, vision rehabilitation therapists, O&M specialists, and low vision professionals, as well as others in the field of blindness can work toward enhancing skills for independence in older adults with visual impairments. Theories of adult learning drive the teaching methods of these professionals. Some of the concepts of adult learning include the following premises (Conti, 2009):

- Adult learning is about problem solving.
- Adults learn when there is a need and readiness to learn.
- Adults become more self-directed and independent with age and experience.
- Intrinsic motivation to learn is the primary motivator for adults.

Understanding and utilizing these principles is crucial to creating an environment in which adults can learn through rehabilitation. Sidebar 7.7 provides specific suggestions for putting these principles into practice with adult learners in general and with those who are visually impaired specifically. Other important factors to consider are that understanding theories of motivation and goal setting can assist anyone teaching adults new skills through rehabilitation (McInerney, Walker, & Liem, 2011; Poulsen, Ziviani, Kotaniemi, & Law, 2014). Instruments such as Assessing the Learning Strategies of Adults (ATLAS) (Conti, 2009) can be used to understand how an individual prefers to approach learning.

SUMMARY

Helping older adults with visual impairments develop and integrate specific O&M and adaptive daily living skills, in combination with supportive social networks, confidence, and a greater appreciation for achieved independence and activity, may greatly enhance their overall life satisfaction. This chapter has presented research to identify critical aspects of life satisfaction for older people with vision loss and provided suggestions for how O&M specialists and other professionals can help older adults tackle barriers in daily living that can ultimately affect their life satisfaction.

SIDEBAR 7.7

Strategies to Assist Adult Learning

Research has shown that adults learn differently from children, and theories of adult learning cite a variety of factors that motivate adults to learn better, some of which are listed here:

LEARNING STRATEGIES FOR ALL ADULTS

- Ensure that curriculum is client-centered and directed.
- Provide feedback to motivate learning.
- Assist adult clients to reach their own conclusions when problem solving.
- It is best when actual needs are the motivators for problem solving. Hypothetical situations may not motivate an adult learner; learning is most effective when relevant to a client's personal situation.
- Learning should be targeted to realistic goals.
- Information to assist learning is best presented in appropriate formats.
- The most effective learning environment is one where the client feels free to ask for help and to ask questions.
- The instructor and adult learner can work collaboratively with shared responsibility for outcomes.
- Adults learn in many ways, and there can be multiple solutions to real-world problems that the learner is exploring.

Older adults with visual impairments may have different needs in the learning process:

LEARNING STRATEGIES FOR THE OLDER ADULT WITH VISION LOSS

- Plan and sequence lessons based on successes; establish further goals for community integration after, or alongside, achievements in independence.
- Recognize the value of peer support while learning new, adaptive skills.
- Acknowledge the role of grief in the learning process, and provide resources for emotional support.
- Recognize that those with vision loss have proved to be faster at processing auditory information than their sighted peers, and utilize this knowledge in teaching.

Source: Adapted from Fone, S. (2006). Effective supervision for occupational therapists: The development and implementation of an information package. *Australian Occupational Therapy Journal 53*, 277–283; Goswami, U. (2004). Neuroscience and education. *British Journal of Educational Psychology, 74*, 1–14.

LEARNING ACTIVITIES

1. Interview an older adult with vision loss about how his or her visual impairment has affected his or her activities of daily living.

2. Using Conti's (2009) Assessing the Learning Strategies of Adults (ATLAS), identify your personal learning strategies.

3. In your place of employment, review emergency preparedness procedures to determine if they are current, comprehensive, and appropriate for older adults with visual impairments. Revise if necessary.

References

Academy for Certification of Vision Rehabilitation and Education Professionals. (2014). *Orientation and mobility specialist certification handbook.* Tucson, AZ: Author.

Academy for Certification of Vision Rehabilitation and Education Professionals. (2015). *ACVREP certification applications.* Tucson, AZ: Author. Retrieved from http://www.acvrep.org/ascerteon/control/certifications

Belsky, J. (1999). *The psychology of aging: Theory, research, and interventions* (3rd ed.). Boston: Cengage Learning.

Binns, A., Bunce, C., Dickinson, C., Harper, R., Tudor-Edwards, R., Woodhouse, M., . . . Margrain, T. (2009, September). *Low vision service outcomes: A systematic review* [Review of the Low Vision Service Model Evaluation Project]. London: Royal National Institute of Blind People. Retrieved from https://www.rnib.org.uk/sites/default/files/LOVESME_lit_review.doc

Boer, L. C., & Withington, D. J. (2004). Auditory guidance in a smoke-filled tunnel. *Ergonomics, 47*(10), 1131–1140.

Bowers, A., & Krader, C. G. (2013). In the driver's seat. *Ophthalmology Times, 38*(2), 53–55.

Carabellese, C., Appollonio, I., Rozzini, R., Bianchetti, A., Frisoni, G. B., Frattola, L., et al. (1993). Sensory impairment and quality of life in a community elderly population. *Journal of the American Geriatrics Society, 41*(4), 401–407.

Carroll, T. J. (1961). *Blindness: What it is, what it does, and how to live with it.* Boston: Little, Brown and Company.

Chou, Y. J., Huang, N., Lee, C. H., Tsai, S. L., Chen, L. S., & Chang, H. J. (2004). Who is at risk of death in an earthquake? *American Journal of Epidemiology, 160*(7), 688–695.

Cicchino, J. B., & McCartt, A. T. (2015). Critical older driver errors in a national sample of serious U.S. crashes. *Accident Analysis & Prevention, 80,* 211–219.

Conti, G. J. (2009). Development of a user-friendly instrument for identifying the learning strategy preferences of adults. *Teaching and Teacher Education, 25*(6), 887–896.

Corn, A. L., & Sacks, S. Z. (1994). The impact of nondriving on adults with visual impairments. *Journal of Visual Impairment & Blindness, 88*(1), 53–68.

Crews, J. E., & Campbell, V. A. (2001). Health conditions, activity limitations, and participation restrictions among older people with visual impairments. *Journal of Visual Impairment & Blindness, 95*(8), 453–467.

Cumming, E., & Henry, W. E. (1961). *Growing old: The process of disengagement.* New York: Basic Books.

Dargent-Molina, P., Hays, M., & Breart, G. (1996). Sensory impairments and physical disability in aged women living at home. *International Journal of Epidemiology, 25*(3), 621–629.

Donorfio, L. K. M., D'Ambrosio, L. A., Coughlin, J. F., & Mohyde, M. (2009). To drive or not to drive, that isn't the question—the meaning of self-regulation among older drivers. *Journal of Safety Research, 40*(3), 221–226.

Duffy, M. A. (2002). *Making life more livable: Simple adaptations for living at home after vision loss.* New York: AFB Press.

Emmons, R. A., & Diener, E. (1985). Factors predicting satisfaction judgements: A comparative examination. *Social Indicators Research, 16*(2), 157–167.

Festinger, L. (1954). A theory of social comparison processes. *Human Relations, 7,* 117–140.

Fonda, G. (1983). Bioptic telescopic spectacle is a hazard for operating a motor vehicle. *Archives of Ophthalmology, 101*(12), 1907–1908.

Fone, S. (2006). Effective supervision for occupational therapists: The development and implementation of an information package. *Australian Occupational Therapy Journal, 53*(4), 277–283.

Frieswijk, N., Buunk, B. P., Steverink, N., & Slaets, J. P. (2004). The interpretation of social comparison and its relation to life satisfaction among elderly people: Does frailty make a difference? *The Journals of Gerontology Series B: Psychological Sciences & Social Sciences, 59*(5), 250–257.

Garcia, P., & McCarthy, M. (1995). *Measuring health: A step in the development of city health profiles.* Copenhagen, Denmark: World Health Organization Regional Office for Europe.

Good, G. A. (2005). *Ageing and vision impairment: Activity, independence and life satisfaction.* Unpublished doctoral thesis, Massey University, Palmerston North, New Zealand. Retrieved from http://muir.massey.ac.nz/bitstream/10179/1542/1/02_whole.pdf

Good, G. A. (2008). Life satisfaction and quality of life of older New Zealanders with and without impaired vision: A descriptive, comparative study. *European Journal of Ageing, 5*(3), 223–231.

Good, G. A., & LaGrow, S. J. (2000). Using peer sampling with older visually impaired adults to set goals for instruction of independent living skills. *RE:view, 32*(3), 132–140.

Good, G. A., Phibbs, S., Williamson, K., & Chambers, P. (2011). *Earthquake and vision impairment: Findings from the Christchurch study.* Unpublished research report, Massey University, Palmerston North, New Zealand.

Good, G. A., Phibbs, S., Williamson, K., & Chambers, P. (2012, February). *Disoriented and immobile: The experiences of people with vision impairment during and after the Christchurch Sept. 2010 earthquake.* Presentation at the 14th International Mobility Conference, Palmerston North, New Zealand.

Goswami, U. (2004). Neuroscience and education. *British Journal of Educational Psychology, 74,* 1–14.

Gowan, M. E., Kirk, R. C., & Sloan, J. A. (2014). Building resiliency: A cross-sectional study examining relationships among health-related quality of life, well-being, and disaster preparedness. *Health and Quality of Life Outcomes, 12,* 85.

Guth, D. A., Rieser, J. J., & Ashmead, D. H. (2010). Perceiving to move and moving to perceive: Control of locomotion by students with vision loss. In W. R. Wiener, R. L. Welsh, & B. B. Blasch (Eds.), *Foundations of orientation and mobility: Vol. I. History and theory* (3rd ed., pp. 3–44). New York: AFB Press.

Hamarat, E., Thompson, D., Aysan, F., Steele, D., Matheny, K., & Simons, C. (2002). Age differences in coping resources and satisfaction with life among middle-aged, young-old, and oldest-old adults. *The Journal of Genetic Psychology, 163*(3), 360–367.

Heidrich, S. M., & Ryff, C. D. (1993). The role of social comparisons processes in the psychological adaptation of elderly adults. *The Journal of Gerontology, 48*(3), 127–136.

Heine, C., & Browning, C. J. (2002). Communication and psychosocial consequences of sensory loss in older adults: Overview and rehabilitation directions. *Disability and Rehabilitation, 24*(15), 763–773.

Horowitz, A., Leonard, R., & Reinhardt, J. P. (2000). Measuring psychosocial and functional outcomes of a group model of vision rehabilitation services for older adults. *Journal of Visual Impairment & Blindness, 94*(5), 328–337.

Horowitz, A., Reinhardt, J. P., Boerner, K., & Travis, L. A. (2003). The influence of health, social support quality and rehabilitation on depression among disabled elders. *Aging & Mental Health, 7*(5), 342–350.

Huss, C. P. (2012). *Prerequisites for rehab specialists involved in the low vision driver education training and assessment process.* Bioptic Driving Network.

Huss, C., & Corn, A. (2004). Low vision driving with bioptics: An overview. *Journal of Visual Impairment & Blindness, 98*(10), 641–653.

LaGrow, S. J. (2004). The effectiveness of comprehensive low vision services for older persons with visual impairments in New Zealand. *Journal of Visual Impairment & Blindness, 98*(11), 679–692.

Lee, H., & Ponchillia, S. V. (2010). Low vision rehabilitation training for working-age adults. In A. L. Corn & J. N. Erin (Eds.), *Foundations of low* vision: *Clinical and functional Perspectives* (2nd ed., pp. 760–798). New York: AFB Press.

Liddle, J., Gustafsson, L., Bartlett, H., & McKenna, K. (2012). Time use, role participation and life satisfaction of older people: Impact of driving status. *Australian Occupational Therapy Journal, 59*(5), 384–392.

Lieberman, L. J., Ponchillia, P. E., & Ponchillia, S. V. (2013). *Physical education and sports for people with visual impairments and deafblindness: Foundations of instruction.* New York: AFB Press.

Luo, G., & Peli, E. (2011). Recording and automated analysis of naturalistic bioptic driving. *Ophthalmic & Physiological Optics, 31*(3), 318–325.

McInerney, D. M., Walker, R. A., & Liem, G. A. D. (Eds.). (2011). Sociocultural theories of learning and motivation: Looking back, looking forward (Vol. 10). In D. M. McInerney (Series Ed.), *Research on sociocultural influences on motivation and learning.* Charlotte, NC: Information Age Publishing.

Marta, M. R., & Geruschat, D. (2004). Equal protection, the ADA, and driving with low vision: A legal analysis. *Journal of Visual Impairment & Blindness, 98*(10), 654–667.

Minto, H., & Butt, I. A. (2004). Low vision devices and training. *Community Eye Health, 17*(49), 6–7.

New Zealand Transport Agency. (2009). *Medical aspects of fitness to drive: A guide for medical practitioners.* Palmerston North, New Zealand: Author.

Orr, A. L. (1991). The psychosocial aspects of aging and vision loss. In N. E. Weber (Ed.), *Vision and aging: Issues in social work practice* (pp. 1–14). Binghamton, NY: Haworth Press.

Orr, A. L., & Rogers, P. A. (2006). *Aging and vision loss: A handbook for families.* New York: AFB Press.

Owsley, C. (2012). Driving with bioptic telescopes: Organizing a research agenda. *Optometry and Vision Science, 89*(9), 1249–1256.

Owsley, C., McGwin, G., Scilley, K., Meek, G. C., Seker, D., & Dyer, A. (2007). Effect of refractive error correction on health-related quality of life and depression in older nursing home residents. *Archives of Ophthalmology, 125*(11), 1471–1477.

Palmer, S. (2005). *Factors which influence the use of low vision aids* [Research report]. Glasgow, UK: Visibility. Retrieved from http://www.visibility.org.uk/what-we-do/research/Low-Vision.pdf

Phibbs, S. R., Woodbury, E., Williamson, K. J., & Good, G. A. (2012). Issues experienced by disabled people following the 2010–2011 Canterbury earthquake series: Evidence based analysis to inform future planning and best practice guidelines for better emergency preparedness. *GNS Science Report, 2012/40,* 53.

Politzer, T. (n.d.). *Implications of acquired monocular vision (loss of one eye).* Valencia, CA: Neuro-Optometric Rehabilitation Association. Retrieved from https://nora.cc/loss-of-one-eye-mainmenu-70.html

Ponchillia, P. E., & Ponchillia, S. V. (1996). *Foundations of rehabilitation teaching with persons who are blind or visually impaired.* New York: AFB Press.

Poulsen, A. A., Ziviani, J., Kotaniemi, K., & Law, M. (2014). 'I think I can': measuring confidence in goal pursuit. *British Journal of Occupational Therapy, 77*(2), 64–66.

Royal National Institute of Blind People. (2015). *Charles Bonnet syndrome.* London: Author. Retrieved from http://www.rnib.org.uk/eyehealth/eyeconditions/conditionsac/Pages/charles_bonnet.aspx

Ryan, E. B., Anas, A. P., Beamer, M., & Bajorek, S. (2003). Coping with age-related vision loss in everyday reading activities. *Educational Gerontology, 29*(1), 37–54.

Schnittker, J. (2007). Look (closely) at all the lonely people: Age and the social psychology of social support. *Journal of Aging and Health, 19*(4), 659–682.

Shipp, M. D., Daum, K. M., Weaver, J. L., Nakagawara, V. B., Bailey, I. L., Good, G. W., . . . Park, W. L. (2000). Motorist vision policy. *Optometry, 71*(7), 449–453.

Stuen, C. (1999). *Family involvement: Maximizing rehabilitation outcomes for older adults with a disability anywhere along the rehabilitation road.* New York: Lighthouse International.

Swagerty, D. L. (1995). The impact of age-related visual impairment on functional independence in the elderly. *Kansas Medicine, 96*(1), 24–26.

Turano, K. A., Broman, A. T., Bandeen-Roche, K., Munoz, B., Rubin, G. S., West, S. K., et al. (2004). Association of visual field loss and mobility performance in older adults: Salisbury eye evaluation study. *Optometry and Vision Science, 81*(5), 298–307.

Warren, M., & Nobles, L. B. (2011). Occupational therapy services for persons with visual impairment. Bethesda, MD: The American Occupational Therapy Association. Retrieved from http://www.aota.org/-/media/Corporate/Files/AboutOT/Professionals/WhatIsOT/PA/Facts/Low%20Vision%20fact%20sheet.pdf

Wilkinson, R., & Marmot, M. (Ed.). (2003). *Social determinants of health: The solid facts* (2nd ed.). Copenhagen, Denmark: World Health Organization.

Williams, R. A., Brody, B. L., Thomas, R. G., Kaplan, R. M., & Brown, S. I. (1998). The psychosocial impact of macular degeneration. *Archives of ophthalmology, 116*(4), 514–520.

World Confederation for Physical Therapy. (2014). Policy statement: Description of physical therapy. London: Author. Retrieved from http://www.wcpt.org/policy/ps-descriptionPT

Ybema, J. F., & Buunk, B. P. (1995). Affective responses to social comparison: A study among disabled individuals. *British Journal of Social Psychology, 34,* 279–292.

CHAPTER 8

Fostering Collaboration among Professionals Serving Older People with Vision Loss

*Rona Pogrund and
Nora Griffin-Shirley*

Some older adults have family support or reside in a community living setting, but others are alone, having lost a spouse or having grown children who live far away. Older adults who live alone must often manage the challenges of aging with little support from others. Each of their stories is different from the next. When an older adult also has a visual impairment, which is one of the most common life changes facing the older person (see Chapter 1), the challenges of aging become even more complex. Vision loss itself can be isolating for many older adults who may lose the ability to drive safely and no longer feel able to manage daily routines or read print on their own.

Lack of independence and potential isolation create the need for collaboration among all those involved in the life of an older adult with a visual impairment. There is no reason for an older adult to be alone or to have to navigate the services and systems that will lead to a higher quality of life without the help of those on his or her rehabilitation team—a team of professionals that may differ depending on the individual's needs and where he or she lives, as discussed in this chapter (see also Chapter 1). It is in the best interest of the client for all professionals who are providing services to collaborate with one another, with the client, and with his or her family members. When each professional works in isolation from others who are also working with the older client, it will result in potential fragmentation (Putnam, 2007). The area of orientation and mobility (O&M) works best in a collaborative service delivery model.

COLLABORATION

Collaboration has been defined as "a process through which different parties who see different aspects of a problem can constructively explore their differences and search for solutions beyond their own limited vision of what is possible" (Gray, 1989, p. 5). Collaboration is not an end in and of itself; it is an ongoing process. It is a process that should continually evolve as the needs of the older adult change and as team members change. Communication and respect are key components in implementing a successful collaboration. Collaboration involves making joint decisions that are focused on what is in the best interest of the older adult. "Collaboration does not occur because of administrative mandate, peer pressure, or political correctness." (Friend, 2000, p. 131) The involvement of a specific number of team members is neither necessarily effective nor a guarantee of quality services. It is the collaboration among team members that increases the likelihood of higher-quality service to the older adult.

COLLABORATIVE TEAM STRATEGIES TO SUPPORT O&M INSTRUCTION

When addressing the issue of independence of an older adult, the O&M specialist is often the leader in defining what this independence may look like, and is the one who may teach specific skills that facilitate this independence. But learning these skills does little good if the older adult only uses and applies the new O&M skills learned during lessons with the O&M specialist present. There must be a commitment on the part of the client to the value of what he or she is learning, as well as support from family members and caregivers as to the importance of the O&M skills learned. To increase the motivation of an older individual, the O&M specialist can use collaborative goal setting, in which the client and specialist agree together on O&M goals (Fazzi & Naimy, 2010), so that the goals are then relevant to the older adult's daily life.

It is not uncommon for older adults with vision loss to learn O&M skills only to be discouraged by family members from using the skills in daily routines. Family members and caregivers may want to do everything for the older adult and do not want to allow him or her to move about independently, even when they have the skills to do so. A similar pattern occurs in community living situations where well-intentioned caregivers and staff members, who frequently have little training and information about visual impairment, tend to lead around older residents with vision loss and jump in to "help" them without waiting to see if they have the ability to handle a situation on their own. Only through collaboration between the O&M specialist, the older adult, family members, and caregivers can these types of situations be avoided so that the older adult can move about and live with dignity and self-sufficiency to the greatest degree possible.

For collaboration to be successful in meeting the needs of the older adult with a visual impairment, the focus needs to constantly be on what is in the best interest of the individual being served. It is just as important for O&M specialists to collaborate with other team members as it is for the O&M specialist to expect the other team members to support the O&M skills he or she is teaching. Sidebar 8.1 provides some suggestions for fostering effective collaboration. For example, the O&M specialist will want to work closely with an older client's medical team regarding any stamina and health problems that need to be considered during an O&M lesson, with the physical therapist regarding adaptations in using a mobility device, with the social worker to know of any social-emotional concerns that may affect O&M lessons, with family members to know what functional needs they feel are important when prioritizing O&M objectives, and, most important, with the older adult to understand the individual's desires and concerns before any O&M lessons can be meaningfully planned.

Working toward "win-win" solutions for any issue encountered by the team is what ultimately benefits the older adult with a visual impairment. Joint problem solving, in which solutions are arrived at in an inclusive fashion, is critical for a collaborative team to be successful. One or more team members may start the problem-solving process but should not predetermine or try to control the outcome for the other team members. Joint problem solving requires mutual respect for all team members. Starting to make changes with the people in a system who are not used to a collaborative model is a process that may take some time. Connecting a new change to something familiar to an individual helps people resistant to change accept it more readily. For example, first offering to incorporate the exercises that the occupational therapist recommends for hand strength at the beginning of each O&M lesson before requesting that O&M techniques be used in an occupational therapy session would begin to introduce the concept of teaming. Modeling effective collaboration for those who are not yet on board is sometimes the most useful

SIDEBAR 8.1

> ## How the O&M Specialist Can Foster Effective Collaboration
>
> The following ideas can promote productive and effective collaboration among team members.
>
> - Use collaborative goal setting to establish O&M goals that are relevant and motivating to the client.
> - Observe other team members working with the client and discuss common concerns and plausible solutions.
> - Actively involve the client in team meetings to establish O&M goals, evaluate progress, and celebrate successes.
> - Involve the client's family members and friends in O&M instruction whenever possible (with permission from the client).
> - Discuss with team members what services need to be direct and which ones need to be consultative to facilitate the client's progress.
> - Model effective communication skills during team meetings and individual conversations with team members, the client, and family members.
> - Allow plenty of time for team meetings.
> - Be creative in communicating with other team members (such as meeting over coffee or communicating via the Internet).
> - Explore the possibility of conducting joint evaluations with other team members.

strategy. Respecting each team member's contributions and expertise, while trying to involve each one in the collaborative process, leads to a higher probability that a collaborative team model will be successful in better meeting the needs of the older adult who is blind or visually impaired.

TEAMS IN DIFFERENT SETTINGS

Collaboration is especially important when the older adult with a visual impairment is working with a variety of professionals with different roles. In this scenario, each specialist has a specific interest in the older adult's well-being, whether it is medical, physical, psychological, logistical, financial, social, or functional. It is not uncommon for many of these professionals to meet individually with a client for their specified purpose and, in many cases, not even communicate with one another. This isolated model of service delivery, based more on a traditional medical model of service delivery, is sometimes a result of the individual receiving services from different systems of providers that may not always interface with each other (Steinman & Moore, 2007). The multiple agencies serving older adults are often in various stages of transition, moving in and out of different funding entities and changing eligibility criteria.

Teams of service providers for older adults exist in different settings, depending on where individuals with vision loss reside and where and from whom they receive services. Some of these settings include public and private rehabilitation centers, nursing homes, assisted living residences, independent living communities, an individual's own home, and hospitals. For example, an older veteran who has a visual impairment may receive in-patient services from a blind rehabilitation center housed in a Veterans Administration hospital run by the U.S. Department of Veterans Affairs. The blind rehabilitation center has a complete rehabilitation team (O&M specialist, vision rehabilitation therapist, low vision therapist) that specializes in evaluation and programming for veterans who are blind or visually impaired. A veteran may also receive services at a Vision Impairment Services Outpatient Rehabilitation (VISOR) program that offers short-term vision rehabilitation.

Some adults with intellectual disabilities have aged in place in state-owned residential facilities, sometimes referred to as supported living centers or human development centers. An O&M specialist may be contracted to provide services to residents of these facilities who have been diagnosed with vision loss. Some individuals with deafblindness and intellectual disabilities were placed in these facilities as children and may not have received O&M training for some time, or ever. With this population, an O&M specialist may be called on to provide training to older residents in the use of unfamiliar assistive technology, to teach routes to newly constructed campus buildings, to provide O&M instruction for the first time, and so on. In this scenario, the O&M specialist will need to work very closely with other team members to learn about the residents' daily routines, functioning levels, behavioral plans, and work routines, as well as the layout of the campus they have to travel across. Most important, the direct-care staff will benefit from learning basic guide and safety techniques and how to ask the residents to move in an appropriate way, especially during emergency drills. It is of utmost importance that the staff learns how to safely move individuals who use wheelchairs.

An older adult with vision loss may also live in a nursing home. His or her nursing home team may consist of a social worker, a nurse, an occupational therapist, a physical therapist, a speech-language pathologist (often referred to as a speech therapist), a music therapist, a physician, an activity director, and several daily caregivers. Recently, the field of low vision rehabilitation services has expanded its services to outpatient clinics in hospitals, outpatient rehabilitation facilities, long-term health care facilities, and nursing homes, in addition to the older person's private home (Watson, 2001). These facilities have teams of professionals, usually including a professional who has been trained to work with older adults with vision loss.

TYPES OF TEAMS THAT WORK WITH THE OLDER ADULT WITH A VISUAL IMPAIRMENT

There are three basic team models used in meeting the needs of individuals with disabilities: multidisciplinary, interdisciplinary, and transdisciplinary.

- *Multidisciplinary*: In this model, a variety of specialized professionals work one-on-one with the individual. Team members seldom communicate, collaborate, or make common agreements, nor do the primary caregivers or the older adult have major input.
- *Interdisciplinary*: This team focuses on the individual's functioning, shares its findings, and develops a joint plan for how best to meet the needs of the older adult.
- *Transdisciplinary*: This model identifies one or a few people who are primarily responsible for direct contact with the individual. This model promotes among team members the pooling and exchange of information, knowledge, and skills that cross and recross traditional boundaries.

In serving the older adult, it is more common for the multidisciplinary team model to be used. In this model, the primary caregivers and the client receive recommendations from separate team members, usually in writing or electronically, that may represent conflicting views, but which the caregiver is expected to interpret and carry out. This model usually includes removing the client from his or her living environment for evaluation, therapy, or appointments, without involving the other team members in the process, and without sharing the rationale and procedures by which the caregiver might complement the work of the specialists. The result can be a very disjointed program (see Sidebar 8.2 for an example of an ineffective team approach).

SIDEBAR 8.2

Example of an Ineffective Team Model

Sarah, an 84-year-old, recently had a stroke and was diagnosed with macular degeneration. She was sent to a short-term care facility for rehabilitation. While there, Sarah was prescribed a wheelchair and received instruction in its use from a physical therapist. A social worker from the care facility arranged for physical therapy services in her home and contacted the state rehabilitation program for older adults who have visual impairments to provide services to Sarah. Jane, an O&M specialist who contracts with the state agency, contacted Sarah to schedule an appointment with her to discuss the O&M services she could provide.

Jane met with Sarah in her home for an evaluation. Jane did not contact Sarah's social worker or her physical therapist to see what her rehabilitation outcomes were. Jane started teaching Sarah how to use a long cane with her wheelchair, an activity contraindicated by the strength-building exercise program that Sarah's physical therapist had developed for her arms and wrists. Sarah had to go to her physician for carpal tunnel issues caused by the use of the long cane. O&M lessons had to be postponed for six weeks to allow Sarah's wrist to heal.

With Sarah's permission, Jane should have contacted Sarah's social worker and her physical therapist to ask about Sarah's rehabilitation goals. Jane could also have scheduled a lesson during the time Sarah's physical therapist was at her home to observe. By sharing information, Sarah, Jane, Sarah's social worker, and her physical therapist could have engaged in collaborative goal setting, thereby preventing Sarah's injury.

The interdisciplinary team model (Hansen, 2008) brings the team together more than the multidisciplinary model, thus reducing fragmentation. The emphasis of the interdisciplinary model is on direct, rather than indirect, services where team members consult with other team members (Cloninger, 2004). However, the primary caregiver's role may still be minimal, and team recommendations may be more ideal than practical because they are based on isolated views of the older adult, not on day-to-day functioning in his or her living environment.

The transdisciplinary team model (Hutchison, 1974), used most often in an educational setting, can also be beneficial in a collaborative team effort when working with adults. In the transdisciplinary model, one or a few people are primarily responsible for direct contact with the individual. Because of the memory issues and physical limitations that some older adults face, the transdisciplinary model may be more beneficial to this population. Thirty or 45 minutes of direct service once or twice a week, or often less frequently, is meaningless to many older adults who have difficulties with generalization and retention of skills. If any real change is to occur, there has to be daily, consistent reinforcement each time a functional opportunity to utilize a skill presents itself. This is possible with a transdisciplinary approach because of the following three important characteristics:

1. Joint team effort—The team of professionals performs the various aspects of program delivery together.
2. Staff development approach—Team members train one another in their particular areas of expertise or share information.
3. Role release—Various professions and disciplines teach others (including caregivers) to implement training procedures and skills that, by tradition, have been considered to be the responsibility of a single profession or discipline. Role release does not imply that professional responsibilities are abdicated; professional accountability is not relinquished in the transdisciplinary approach. Team members must remain accountable for what they teach others and for how well the skills are obtained by the client.

The transdisciplinary approach may seem more difficult and time consuming to some professionals. In reality, if a specialist serves in more of a consultative role in training others who can implement a particular expertise on a daily basis, as opposed to performing all direct instruction with an older adult on a limited basis, the specialist may be able to reach more clients and have an greater overall impact, and the client will have greater chances for generalization and utilization of skills.

For example, if the O&M specialist wants an older client living in a community living facility to utilize cane skills, which are being taught during O&M lessons once a week for an hour, it is critical that all staff and caregivers at the residence be taught what cane skills the individual should be using so that these skills can be reinforced throughout the day as the client goes to and from the dining hall, to activities within and outside of the building, to the doctor's office, and so on. It is the O&M specialist's job to continually monitor how skills are being implemented and generalized and to intervene if necessary. Integrating skills learned from different specialists within daily routines through team support is a better use of any specialist's expertise than isolated instruction shared only in a written report. When team members share power and invest in the collaborative process, the team is stronger and the client benefits.

ROLES AND RESPONSIBILITIES OF TEAM MEMBERS

Generally, the rehabilitation team consists of the older adult with vision loss, family members, and medical and rehabilitation professionals. To work effectively, the team members must collaborate with one another and share their expertise.

The primary member of the team is the older client with vision loss. In conjunction with the team members, older adults decide their needs, what assistive devices they will use and when and where they will use them, when instruction is convenient, and the like. Usually, a contract that outlines the specifics of a rehabilitation plan is developed by the rehabilitation counselor, with input from the client. It is imperative that older adults with vision loss realize they are ultimately responsible for carrying out their own rehabilitation plan with support from their family members (Corn & Lusk, 2010).

Family members are crucial players in the rehabilitation of older adults with vision loss. Their involvement can improve the quality of life for their loved ones. Family members can contribute to the rehabilitation process in a variety of ways, including the following:

- Provide input about how the client functions and reinforce new skills learned to help the client complete common activities of daily living.
- Encourage the use of strategies for coping with vision loss suggested by professionals.
- Help make environmental modifications to the client's home.
- Assist with transportation to low vision clinic examinations, grocery stores, and doctor appointments.
- Advocate for the client to receive high quality services if the client is unable to advocate for him- or herself.
- Treat their loved one with respect and dignity as he or she copes with vision loss.

Medical and vision rehabilitation personnel are also part of the team. Medical personnel may include primary care physicians, ophthalmologists, optometrists specializing in low vision, nurses, physical therapists, occupational therapists, counselors, psychologists, caseworkers, nurse's aides, nursing assistants, and speech-language pathologists. The vision rehabilitation team may consist of low vision therapists, vision rehabilitation therapists, O&M specialists, social workers, and assistive technology professionals. Additional team members may include recreational therapists, audiologists, and physicians in various specialties (such as orthopedists and neurologists) depending on the physical, mental, and emotional needs of the individual. (Sidebar 8.3 provides a list of team members and examples of how they may be involved in O&M instruction.) In general, medical professionals care for the overall health and well-being of the older person with vision loss, provide instruction in disease management, and make referrals to specialists like ophthalmologists for eye care. The vision rehabilitation team evaluates, develops, and delivers an instructional program and suggests assistive technology to improve the independence of the older adult.

The roles and responsibilities of team members working with older adults with vision loss overlap. For example, overlap exists between the roles of the nurse and the primary care physician when it comes to offering public awareness about vision loss among older adults, education to the patient and his or her family about the patient's eye condition, and referrals for the patient to a variety of services. Watson (2001) identifies numerous services primary care physicians and geriatricians (physicians who specialize in care for people 65 and older and who have additional training in the medical, social, and psychological issues of older adults) can provide to patients with low vision, including the following:

- visual acuity evaluation
- contrast sensitivity function evaluation
- referral to a low vision clinic and vision rehabilitation professionals
- identification (with the patient) of rehabilitation goals
- reinforcement of the goals that have been met after the patient has received training
- referral to counseling and support groups to adjust to vision loss
- explanation—to a patient and the patient's family—of how a patient's vision loss affects what he or she can see
- increasing public awareness about vision loss among older adults

SIDEBAR 8.3

Roles and Responsibilities of Rehabilitation Team Members in O&M Training

ASSISTIVE TECHNOLOGY PROFESSIONAL

Evaluates, recommends, and trains the older adult in the use of assistive technology needed to improve his or her daily functioning (Rehabilitation Engineering and Assistive Technology Society of North America, 2014). An assistive technology professional who is also a seating and mobility specialist may work closely with a physical therapist and an O&M specialist when assisting an older adult in selecting the optimal positioning in a wheelchair to use his or her vision effectively.

AUDIOLOGIST

Specializes in hearing and balance and diagnostics and remediation of the auditory system. An audiologist can change the settings of a hearing aid to allow an older adult to hear traffic and other ambient sounds while on O&M lessons.

CARETAKER (AIDE, NURSING ASSISTANT)

Implements the physician's directives for medical care and supports and reinforces the adaptive strategies older adults use to cope with vision loss, such as cueing an older adult to use appropriate guide techniques in his or her home.

LOW VISION THERAPIST

Provides instruction for older adults with vision loss in visual efficiency skills and the use of prescribed optical devices (like a telescope the older client may use to see the WALK/DON'T WALK sign at an intersection).

ORIENTATION AND MOBILITY SPECIALIST

Provides direct and consultative services leading to systematic orientation to, and safe movement within, clients' living and working environments.

VISION REHABILITATION THERAPIST

Evaluates, plans, and provides direct instruction in communication and daily living skills for older adults with vision loss. For example, the vision rehabilitation therapist may work closely with an older adult on money management for an O&M grocery shopping lesson (Ponchillia & Ponchillia, 1996).

(continued)

SIDEBAR 8.3 *(continued)*

COUNSELOR OR PSYCHOLOGIST

Provides therapeutic counseling and administers tests to determine intellectual function, adjustment to vision loss, and personality issues. To alleviate stress due to O&M lessons, for example, a counselor may suggest that an older adult use deep breathing exercises.

IN-HOME ATTENDANT

Supports older adults as they learn to use assistive devices and reinforces their correct usage. Cares for the daily needs of older adults as requested by medical and rehabilitation professionals and family members. An in-home attendant may, if present to observe O&M lessons, reinforce the use of O&M skills while an older person is walking around his or her home.

OCCUPATIONAL THERAPIST

Trains and retrains older adults in motor skills to independently complete activities of daily living. May have training in assessing visual problems, making effective adaptations, and conducting assessments collaboratively with the O&M specialist or vision rehabilitation therapist. An occupational therapist, an older individual, and an O&M specialist may decide together what environmental modifications in the older person's home are appropriate to make it easier for him or her to get around inside and outside the house.

OPHTHALMOLOGIST

Specializes in the care of the eye and the visual system and advocates for the prevention of eye disease (Corn & Lusk, 2010; Ponchillia & Ponchillia, 1996). With the older adult's permission, an O&M specialist may provide an O&M evaluation report to a client's ophthalmologist for review.

OPTOMETRIST

Works with the functioning rather than the pathology of the eye. Measures refraction, prescribes and fits corrective lenses, and prescribes optical devices (with specialized training in low vision). This professional may prescribe optical devices to older adults with vision loss that can be used to improve their travel skills in the community. See Chapter 7 for more information on the use of optical devices.

LOW VISION SPECIALIST

Conducts clinical low vision evaluations and prescribes appropriate near and distance optical devices. The low vision specialist is usually an optometrist or ophthalmologist who has special training in caring for people with low vision. The O&M specialist may accompany an older adult to an appointment to assist in the discussion of the person's travel needs and what devices may work well in certain environments.

PHYSIATRIST

Specializes in helping patients restore function and overcome physical limitations. At the request of an O&M specialist, a physiatrist can, for example, develop a specific program of exercises to strengthen the hand and arm used by the older adult to grip his or her cane.

PHYSICAL THERAPIST

"Provides therapy to change the level of physical functioning of older people" (Freburger & Holmes, 2005, p. 20). The physical therapist can, for example, teach an older adult who has had two knee replacements how to use a one-handed support device while the O&M specialist instructs the client in the use of the support device and a long cane.

PHYSICIAN

Cares for and monitors the health of older adult patients. The increased physical activity involved in O&M training may create a need to adjust medications. For example, people with diabetes will need to closely monitor blood-sugar levels, and medications may need to be adjusted for O&M lessons. Before beginning O&M training, older adults should check with their physicians.

RECREATIONAL THERAPIST

Directs and organizes fitness activities, dramatics, games, arts and crafts in residential facilities to assist patients in developing interpersonal relationships, socializing effectively, and developing the confidence needed to participate in group activities (*Directory of Occupational Titles,* 2003). Consultation with O&M specialists can facilitate maximum benefit from both programs.

SPEECH-LANGUAGE PATHOLOGIST

Evaluates and treats speech, language, cognitive communication, and swallowing disorders. A speech-language pathologist can help an older individual with speech difficulties resulting from a stroke, to communicate his or her needs effectively during travel.

SOCIAL WORKER

Assesses clients' needs and coordinates services to promote their independence in their home and in the community. During a counseling session, a social worker may work closely with an older client's family members to discuss their feelings about the client traveling independently on public transportation, if, for example, he or she has never been on a bus before.

Houde and Huff (2003) suggest that the role of gerontological nurses is complex when working with older adults with vision loss. Their "role includes increasing public awareness, early disease detection, support for older adults with vision impairment and their family members, providing education about vision loss and resources, political and patient advocacy, and research" (Houde & Huff, 2003, p. 32). Research exploring the efficacy of interventions by medical personnel, their roles, and the resources provided for this population is greatly needed.

One of the issues that older adults with vision loss and their families face is the lack of referral from medical personnel for vision rehabilitation services. Corn and Lusk (2010) state: "primary care providers do not routinely make referrals to educational and rehabilitation personnel in nonmedical facilities. There is sometimes a similar lack of coordination between allied health care providers, such as occupational therapists who perform a variety of vision rehabilitation services" (p. 26). This lack of referral increases the amount of time older adults with vision loss are at home without help for a deteriorating visual condition, which can lead to depression. Appropriate referral will help ameliorate both of these problems. Effective collaboration increases the chances that older adults with vision loss will receive targeted instructional programming that will help them adjust to their visual conditions.

SUCCESSFUL TEAMS AND BARRIERS TO COLLABORATION

There are certain factors that are common to most successful teams, including mutual respect, trust, commitment to planning, and a common philosophy (Barnes & Turner, 2001; Mastropieri et al., 2005). According to Friend and Cook (2012), successful collaboration is

- voluntary,
- requires parity among team members,
- based on mutual goals,
- depends on shared responsibility for participation and decision making,
- requires sharing of resources, and
- requires accountability for outcomes.

Communication among all team members is central to a collaborative team model. Some of the basic rules of effective communication—such as being polite when interacting with others, really listening, using supportive communication strategies, and having a sense of humor—are essential for building the rapport needed for developing successful collaboration. Without this necessary rapport among all team members, it is hard to work constructively as a collaborative team. Often teams will include some members who do not easily connect because of different personality styles, varying communication approaches, or differences in philosophy, but it is still important to reach out to those team members with the focus on what is best for the individual the team serves. Showing interest in the lives of other team members and trying to understand their expertise and perspectives can build bridges between team members who may not automatically connect. Sometimes, building rapport can start with something as simple as an offer to have coffee together or get together for lunch. Trying to find time to interact in the midst of everyone's busy schedules takes creativity, but most professionals working with older adults—whether in a medical, rehabilitation, community living, or home setting—still have to take a break and have lunch. Even though the byproduct of a successful collaborative effort may be that the team members feel better about their interactions with one another and are more satisfied with their job roles, it is important to remember that this outcome is not the primary focus of the collaborative effort. The purpose of any collaboration is to ensure that the service delivery system provides the best services possible to the older adult with a visual impairment (Friend, 2000). It is also important to realize that collaborative skills do not come naturally to all people, and that some people need to learn such skills in order to work in a team environment.

Some collaborative strategies that help develop a sense of working as a team and trust among team members include the following (Knackendoffel, 2005):

- showing respect for other team members
- valuing the other team member's expertise and contribution
- exhibiting trustworthiness through your actions (for example, show up when you say you will and follow through on any agreements you make)
- recognizing the other person's stressors related to his or her job (for example, a large number and great diversity of older adults to serve, significant amounts of paperwork, overtime, low pay)
- maintaining confidentiality
- changing your communication style to better connect with other team members

- avoiding getting too locked into your own ideas in case they are not received well by other team members

Sometimes, existing barriers to successful collaboration and teamwork need to be acknowledged and addressed in order to move forward. (See Sidebar 8.4 for a summary of some challenges to collaborative teams.) When professionals work for different entities with different fiscal systems, organizational barriers can make collaboration difficult. Health care, social services, and rehabilitation services are often under varying public and private organizations that have different accountability requirements and funding sources. Although service providers from all of these systems may be working with the same older adult with a visual impairment, it can be hard for them to collaboratively integrate their services. Each of these systems may have a different culture from the other and may adhere to a different team model (for instance, a multidisciplinary medical model versus a transdisciplinary social-service model).

There can also be differing professional values among team members. Each specialist may relate more to the other professionals in his or her area of expertise rather than to someone outside his or her specialty area. Vision professionals belong to one professional organization, physical and occupational

---

SIDEBAR 8.4

Challenges to Collaboration

Factors that serve as barriers to successful collaboration include the following:

- Professionals work for different entities with different fiscal systems.
- Service delivery systems may have varying cultures and different team models.
- Team members have differing professional values.
- Professionals belong to different professional organizations and attend their own conferences with their own jargon.
- Team members have personality differences.
- Team members are under time constraints.
- Team members have a fear of collaboration.
- Team members are concerned about their social roles and who is perceived as having the most power.

therapists belong to others, and medical professionals to yet another group. Each specialist typically attends his or her own professional conferences and training rather than jointly attending with other team members from a different professional area. The lack of shared professional language and philosophies from different disciplines can also be a barrier to productive teams (Robinson & Buly, 2007).

Personal barriers also exist that can inhibit a positive collaborative effort. The personality differences mentioned earlier make some people more comfortable than others in working as a team. Different personality styles may have different impacts on effective collaboration. Some people are extroverts who like working closely with groups of people while others are introverts who prefer to work on their own.

Some team members may seem to be resistant to collaboration. Many people who are resistant to the collaborative process feel this way because it involves change, and change is hard for many people. Some people are comfortable doing things as they have always been done, and they can find many reasons—some that they may share and others that they may not—for not wanting to participate in a collaborative team effort. Some resistors will verbally agree to collaborate but then just not do it, or they will procrastinate in carrying out the steps that need to be taken and thus show more passive resistance.

Time is the most frequent reason people feel they cannot collaborate. They feel they are just too busy to be bothered to work in a team. They think it takes too much time to develop the needed relationships, to train one another in their expertise, and to observe and monitor others who should be implementing skills they teach. According to Friend (2000), "By acknowledging the time demands of collaboration, it becomes a legitimate professional responsibility and moves away from being an invisible but pressing expectation" (p. 131). For successful collaboration to occur, time needs to be set aside and prioritized for scheduling the development of the collaborative team process. The lead for such scheduling typically has to come from supervisors and administrators who value the collaborative process even if it necessitates working with leaders of other service delivery systems to facilitate the collaboration. O&M specialists can request more time for team meetings from their supervisors.

There are other common reasons for avoiding collaboration. One professional may fear that if he or she collaborates with others, the other team members might think that they can do his or her job as well as he or she can. This fear may stem from a lack of confidence on the part of the professional who is afraid to let go of any of his or her expertise. He or she may be resistant to releasing his or her role for fear that his or her job will become obsolete. Another issue that serves as a barrier to successful collaboration is the concern about the social roles of the team members: who on the team is perceived as possessing the most power either because of his or her position, salary, employer, or other factor? A true collaborative team does not look at fellow team members in this way. In a collaborative team, all members contribute to the well-being of the older adult, so all team members are considered valuable, including family members and other caregivers; in fact, they are often the most valuable members of the team since they spend the most time with the older adult who is blind or visually impaired.

Another potential barrier to effective collaboration results from the fact that roles and team members change often, which can make accountability and responsibility difficult to track. There is a strong push for accountability among all social services today (Lackey, 2006; Ludowise, 2004), and if there is too much collaboration in serving the older adult, the services provided may overlap and it may appear difficult to determine who is actually responsible for which outcomes. With each professional being expected to provide accountability for meeting specific goals and objectives for the client in his or her particular area of expertise, there may be a concern as to how he or she will monitor achievement if too many others on the team are helping to meet the older adult's objectives. In reality, time that is devoted to collaboration should lead to results that can be documented for accountability purposes. If team members keep changing, it makes it harder to maintain continuity and requires that new relationships and communication systems be established with each new team member, thus possibly inhibiting the team process already in place.

SUMMARY

Many older adults who are blind or visually impaired also have additional medical, physical, social, and emotional challenges that require a team of professionals to address. For O&M goals to be realized, this team must collaborate successfully. O&M specialists working with older clients with vision loss can assume leadership roles in modeling effective collaboration for other team members. When team members use an effective team model and practice good communication skills, collaborative goal setting, and strategies that foster collaboration, older adults with vision loss benefit by receiving better, more cohesive services, leading to greater independence in travel. This independence can lead to a better quality of life for older adults with visual impairments.

LEARNING ACTIVITIES

1. Review the strategies for effective collaboration listed in Sidebar 8.1. Discuss with another O&M specialist the strategies he or she uses to facilitate effective collaboration when working with a team serving an older adult with vision loss. Compare those strategies to the strategies listed in the sidebar. Identify what worked well with an older population.

2. Obtain permission from the administration of a rehabilitation center serving older adults with vision loss to observe a team meeting. Note what type of team model was used, the type of communication styles team members exhibited, and the challenges the team faced.

3. Interview other O&M specialists and other rehabilitation personnel about their experiences being part of a team that delivers rehabilitation training to older adults with vision loss. Develop a list of techniques that facilitated collaboration among the team members.

4. Discuss with an older adult with vision loss his or her experiences when meeting with his or her service team. From this conversation, identify who was on the team and the role each team member played. Did the older adult feel he or she was central to the team's efforts? If so, what behaviors did team members demonstrate to make the older adult feel this way. If not, why not?

References

Barnes, K. J., & Turner, K. D. (2001). Team collaborative practices between teachers and occupational therapists. *American Journal of Occupational Therapy, 55*(1), 83–89.

Cloninger, C. J. (2004). Designing collaborative educational services. In F. P. Orelove, D. Sobsey, & R. K. Silberman (Eds.), *Educating children with multiple disabilities: A collaborative approach* (4th ed., pp. 1–29). Baltimore, MD: Paul H. Brookes Publishing Co.

Corn, A. L., & Lusk, K. E. (2010). Perspectives on low vision. In A. L. Corn & J. N. Erin (Eds.), *Foundations of low vision: Clinical and functional perspectives* (2nd ed., pp. 3–34). New York: AFB Press.

Directory of Occupational Titles. (2003). *Recreational therapist*. Retrieved September 24, 2014, from http://www.occupationalinfo.org/07/076124014.html

Fazzi, D. L., & Naimy, B. J. (2010). Teaching orientation and mobility to school-age children. In W. R. Wiener, R. L. Welsh, & B. B. Blasch (Eds.), *Foundations of orientation and mobility: Vol. II. Instructional strategies and practical applications* (3rd ed., pp. 208–262). New York: AFB Press.

Freburger, J. K., & Holmes, G. M. (2005). Physical therapy use by community-based older people. *Physical Therapy, 85*(1), 19–33.

Friend, M. (2000). Myths and misunderstandings about professional collaboration. *Remedial and Special Education, 21*, 130–132, 160.

Friend, M., & Cook, L. (2012). *Interactions: Collaboration skills for school professionals*. New York: Pearson.

Gray, B. (1989). *Collaborating: Finding common ground for multiparty problems*. San Francisco: Jossey-Bass Inc.

Hansen, J. C. (2008). Community and in-home models. *American Journal of Nursing, 108*(9), 69–72.

Houde, S. C., & Huff, M. H. (2003). Age-related vision loss in older adults. A challenge for gerontological nurses. *Journal of Gerontological Nursing, 29*(4), 25–33.

Hutchison, D. A. (1974). A model for transdisciplinary staff development. In *A nationally organized collaborative program for the provision of comprehensive services to atypical infants and their families* (Technical Report No. 8). New York: United Cerebral Palsy Association.

Knackendoffel, E. A. (2005). Collaborative teaming in the secondary school. *Focus on Exceptional Children, 37*(5), 1–16.

Lackey, J. F. (2006). *Accountability in social services: The culture of the paper program*. New York: The Haworth Press.

Ludowise, C. (2004). Accountability in social service contracting: The state action doctrine and beyond. *Journal of Health and Human Services Administration, 27*(3), 304–330.

Mastropieri, M. A., Scruggs, T. E., Graetz, J., Norland, J., Gardizi, W., & McDuffie, K. (2005). Case studies in co-teaching in the content areas: Successes, failures, and challenges. *Intervention in School and Clinic, 40*(5), 260–270.

Ponchillia, P. E., & Ponchillia, S. V. (1996). *Foundations of rehabilitation teaching with persons who are blind or visually impaired*. New York: AFB Press.

Putnam, M. (2007). Moving from separate to crossing aging and disability service networks. In M. Putnam (Ed.), *Aging and disability: Crossing network lines* (pp. 5–17). New York: Springer.

Rehabilitation Engineering and Assistive Technology Society of North America. (2014). *ATP: Become a certified assistive technology professional*. Retrieved from http://www.resna.org/get-certified/atp/atp

Robinson, L., & Buly, M. R. (2007). Breaking the language barrier: Promoting collaboration between general and special educators. *Teacher Education Quarterly, 34*(3), 83–94.

Steinman, B. A., & Moore, J. E. (2007). Collaborative activities by state older blind independent living programs [Research report]. *Journal of Visual Impairment & Blindness, 101*(11), 715–720.

Watson, G. R. (2001). Low vision in the geriatric population: Rehabilitation and management. *Journal of the American Geriatrics Society, 49*(3), 317–330.

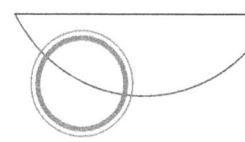

Epilogue
Current and Emerging Issues for O&M Service Provision

Nora Griffin-Shirley

This book has described the various aspects of providing orientation and mobility (O&M) services for older adults with vision loss. Before concluding, however, it would be important to mention the issues and challenges currently faced by this practice, including the following:

- Lack of awareness by professionals and older adults of O&M services and how to access them.
- Insufficiency of third-party reimbursement for services by public funding.
- Lack of services that account for language and cultural differences.
- Lack of services that address the environmental and geographic aspects unique to older adults with vision loss.
- Increase of incidence of medical conditions such as Alzheimer's and diabetes.
- Shortage of qualified personnel to provide services to older adults with vision loss.
- Few standardized assessment tools to measure efficacy of O&M training.
- Relative lack of evidence-based research addressing efficacy of teaching techniques and strategies.

In addition, the negative attitudes of older adults, families, and society toward visual impairments play a crucial role in the provision of O&M services (see Chapter 1 for more information concerning this topic).

These issues have been cited in various pieces of legislation (such as the Rehabilitation Act of 1973 and the Older Americans Act of 1965) by organizations serving older adults who are visually impaired (such as the American

Foundation for the Blind, the National Federation of the Blind, and the American Council of the Blind), and in documents concerning older adults with vision loss, such as the National Agenda on Vision and Aging (Orr, Scott, & Rogers, 2005). Spearheaded by the American Foundation for the Blind, the National Agenda on Vision and Aging was developed in 1998 by the National Aging and Vision Network, a group of agencies and professionals serving older adults with vision loss. This document provides professionals with seven goals for older adults to be fully included in society (Orr & Rogers, 2001). Avenues for addressing the challenges mentioned by these entities include the following:

- research into best practices in working with older adults
- increased funding for services and infrastructure
- expanding personnel preparation for O&M instruction to older adults with visual impairments
- encouraging self-advocacy among older adults with vision loss
- increased public education about O&M instruction for older adults
- certification of professionals working with older adults with visual impairments

Table 9.1 summarizes the challenges and the approaches to addressing them that are discussed in this chapter.

RESEARCH

As early as 1980, De l'Aune discussed the need for O&M practitioners to engage in research to fill "the gaps in our present knowledge of mobility" (De l'Aune, 1980, p. 661) because they have access to potential research participants, while Wall Emerson and De l'Aune (2010) mentioned the ability of O&M specialists to observe their students and clients in many different situations. Similarly, Wiener and Welsh (1980) suggested that practitioners "must do more writing and research than they have done in the past, and the profession must stimulate and reward such activity" (p. 644). Wall Emerson and De l'Aune (2010) are still advocating for practitioners to conduct research.

The National Eye Institute (NEI; 2012) has identified a number of areas for future research directly related to O&M in their report, *Vision Research: Needs, Gaps, and Opportunities*, including the following:

TABLE 9.1 Response to Challenges to the Provision of O&M Services for Older Adults with Vision Loss

Challenges to the Provision of O&M Services for Older Adults with Vision Loss	Suggested Responses for O&M Specialists
Relative lack of evidence-based research addressing efficacy of teaching techniques and strategies. Few standardized assessment tools to measure efficacy of orientation and mobility training.	• Design and conduct studies that look at teaching strategies routinely used by O&M specialists with the older adults they instruct. Disseminate results at conferences and through journals. • Volunteer as participants in research projects. • Join teams that are designing instruments to measure efficacy and outcomes.
Insufficiency of third-party reimbursement for services by public funding. Shortage of qualified personnel to provide services to older adults with vision loss.	• Become active in professional organizations, agencies for people who are visually impaired, and consumer groups who are involved in changing the laws for licensure of O&M specialists and for obtaining insurance funding for O&M services. • Teach clients and their family members how to advocate for increased services, including through the licensure of O&M specialists and for insurance coverage for O&M services.
Lack of services that account for language and cultural differences. Lack of services that address environmental and geographic aspects unique to older adults with vision loss.	• Advocate for and provide instruction that accounts for language and cultural differences by using an interpreter and learning about clients' cultures. • Learn about the range of settings clients with vision loss live in and consider how these environments affect, support, or challenge clients' O&M.
Increased incidence of medical conditions such as Alzheimer's and diabetes.	• Engage in professional development activities concerning common medical conditions affecting the older adult population. • Offer training on this topic to other O&M specialists through conference presentations, webinars, newsletters, and journal articles.

(continued)

TABLE **9.1** (*continued*)

Challenges to the Provision of O&M Services for Older Adults with Vision Loss	Suggested Responses for O&M Specialists
Lack of awareness by professionals and older adults of O&M services and how to access them.	• Provide local aging and medical networks with information concerning O&M training and vision rehabilitation services.
Negative attitudes of older adults, families, and society toward visual impairments.	• Encourage clients and their families to receive counseling and join support groups. • Provide O&M lessons where clients can measure their success.
Confusion over which professionals should provide O&M training to older adults with vision loss.	• Advocate for licensure and certification of professionals who provide O&M training. • Become involved in efforts to define the roles and responsibilities of aging, medical, and rehabilitation professionals who provide services to older adults with vision loss.

- the contribution of nonvisual cues to spatial cognition
- the use of cognitive maps in learning strategies and the effect of age
- the development and validation of vision tests for activities of daily living and tests for evaluation of complex intensive behavior (such as mobility and driving)
- the creation of assistive technology and applications related to mobile phones and global positioning systems
- the use of eccentric viewing for navigation
- the use of visual prosthesis for completion of mobility tasks

The NEI (2012) has also suggested that researchers explore how comorbid conditions affect individuals as they age. Seeking answers to the following questions helps serve older adults with these conditions:

1. How does Alzheimer's affect the spatial organization and cognitive mapping ability areas in the brain of an older person with a visual impairment?

2. What are the most effective interventions O&M specialists can implement with individuals with Alzheimer's and vision loss to help them remain oriented and travel to where they want to go?
3. If an older person with a visual impairment has multiple conditions such as diabetes, a hearing impairment, orthopedic impairment, and dementia, what team model is best to use?
4. How can the aging, medical, and rehabilitation fields collaborate to ensure these older individuals receive all the services they require at the appropriate times so they can remain as independent as possible in their current living environments?
5. What are the roles of the professionals who work with this population?
6. How do we, as professionals, come to a consensus when our roles blur?

In addition, the NEI suggests specific research topics aimed at improving rehabilitation and public health, such as testing of rehabilitation models and exploring the effectiveness of rehabilitation approaches. In the area of low vision and mobility, Virgili and Rubin (2010) advocate for more research to be conducted on the effectiveness of different types of training for people with low vision and to decide on standardized measurements for mobility performance to use in future studies. Their suggestion is based on their review of the literature and subsequent evaluation of studies looking at the effects of O&M training on physical exercise of adults with low vision, where only two studies were found. It is reasonable to assume their recommendation could also extend to the effects of O&M training for older adults with vision loss.

Yeung, LaGrow, Towers, Alpass, and Stephens (2011) stress investigating "a broad array of psychological, social, and/or physical variables as mediators of the relationships between the ability to get around and QOL [quality of life]" (p. 18) in individuals with visual impairments. Two recent studies have shown a connection between the ability to get around and the quality of life perception by people who have difficulty seeing (LaGrow, Alpass, Stephens, & Towers, 2011; Yeung et al., 2011). Therefore, O&M training is an important component of the rehabilitation process for older adults with vision loss. However, in *Vision Rehabilitation for Elderly Individuals with Low Vision or Blindness* (Agency for Healthcare Research and Quality, 2004), it is reported that "the effectiveness (or lack of effectiveness) of orientation and mobility training has yet to be demonstrated by a well-designed study that has utilized validated instruments to measure outcome" (p. 97).

FUNDING

Farquhar, Lowe, and Campbell (2007) identify trends in funding in the aging field that include areas relevant to O&M, such as building community capacity to support aging and age-friendly communities (Plouffe & Kalache, 2010), developing a more comprehensive and flexible concept of long-term care, and expanding community-based care. The field of O&M needs to become familiar with these funding trends and strategically plan how to interface with funders interested in aging and vision loss projects. Many of the trends are already used with client-centered and family-based models.

The World Health Organization (2007) conducted a study with 1,485 older adults over the age of 60, 250 caregivers, and 515 service providers, to identify what constitutes an urban area that promotes mobility, physical accessibility, service proximity, security, affordability, and inclusiveness. One hundred and fifty-eight focus groups were conducted in 33 cities globally. The participants were asked to identify positive and negative features of cities, focusing on outdoor spaces and public buildings, housing, social participation, respect and social inclusion, civic participation and employment, communication and information, community support, and health services. One of the major results was the need for urban planners to stress enablement, not disablement, when designing city features for older city dwellers (Plouffe & Kalache, 2010; World Health Organization, 2007). Adequate funding is needed to make the suggested changes to cities in order to promote age-friendly communities.

Licensure of O&M specialists will help justify the third-party reimbursement of O&M services by public funding. For many years the O&M field, rehabilitation agencies, lobbyists, and blindness consumer groups have been actively pursuing licensure in New York, Pennsylvania, and Tennessee (Wiener & Siffermann, 2010). If this goal is achieved, the sources of funding for O&M services to older adults who warrant them will be expanded to health insurance plans. Continued efforts by O&M specialists to change laws for licensure and third-party reimbursement are necessary.

PERSONNEL PREPARATION

Professional development programs focusing on curricula for the provision of O&M instruction to older adults with visual impairments at the preservice and in-service levels need to be expanded to keep pace with the growing number of older adults in the United States (Welsh, 1980). Curricula should also remain current with common medical conditions affecting older adults such as Alzheimer's and diabetes. The fourth goal of the National Agenda on Vision and Aging calls for an increase of qualified professionals—including O&M specialists (Orr & Rogers, 2001; National Aging and Vision Network Work Group, 1999)—to receive high-quality services and for personnel preparation programs to revise their curricula to better address this population. O&M specialists can take advantage of specific training provided through e-learning, webinars, and print materials from in-service training, university personnel preparation programs, and organizations such as the American Foundation for the Blind, American Printing House for the Blind, Association for Education and Rehabilitation of the Blind and Visually Impaired, and Lighthouse International.

ADVOCACY AND EMPOWERMENT

Consumer choice in rehabilitation services is an important component of federal legislation (Orr & Rogers, 2001). Many times older adults may not be accustomed to advocating for services they need such as O&M instruction. To assist them in requesting this instruction, older adults can be taught how to better advocate for themselves. For example, the first goal of the National Agenda on Aging and Vision Loss is "to develop a consumer self-advocacy skills training curriculum" (Orr, Scott, & Rogers, 2005). This topic has been included in many curricula developed for older adults with vision loss and their families. Examples include *Aging and Vision Loss: A Handbook for Families* (Orr & Rogers, 2006) and *Self-Advocacy Skills Training for Older Individuals Who Are Visually Impaired* (Orr & Rogers, 2003). O&M specialists can be proactive in the provision of information to local aging and medical networks concerning O&M services and how to make referrals for this service.

PUBLIC EDUCATION

Public education materials addressing O&M are delivered through television, social media, websites, print materials, blogs, webinars, and lectures. Some public education resources are related solely to O&M, such as "An Introduction to Orientation and Mobility Skills" (Sauerburger, n.d.) on the Vision-Aware website of the American Foundation for the Blind.

Public education programs about O&M services should focus on who is a candidate for O&M instruction, what an O&M program entails, who is qualified to provide this instruction, which entity pays for these services, and how older adults with vision loss can access these services. Targeted information about agencies and providing O&M services to hard-to-reach and high-risk groups (such as Native Americans and Hispanics) needs to be disseminated (Orr, 1998).

CERTIFICATION OF PROFESSIONALS PROVIDING O&M SERVICES

Students in university O&M training usually apply for certification through the Academy for the Certification of Vision Rehabilitation and Education Professionals (ACVREP) and the National Blindness Professionals Certification Board (NBPCB). Continued efforts need to be made to ensure that all professionals providing O&M services to older adults with visual impairments are certified. Other professionals (such as occupational therapists and physical therapists) should also be encouraged to continue to seek training as O&M specialists and to obtain certification through ACVREP or NBPCB.

When serving the older adult population, there are times when the roles and responsibilities among aging and rehabilitation professionals overlap. Respectful and effective dialogue among these professionals will help identify how both fields can determine and meet the O&M needs of older adults with visual impairments. The O&M Division of the Association for the Education and Rehabilitation of the Blind and Visually Impaired has appointed a committee—Best Practice in Collaboration: O&M and OT & PT Scope of Practice—to develop a position paper and to collect data documenting the type of coursework that is required by the licensure organizations for occupational therapists and physical therapists (Associate for Education and Rehabilitation of the Blind and Visually Impaired, 2014).

SUMMARY

When providing O&M services to older adults with visual impairments, certain challenges exist. O&M specialists can be proactive in engaging in activities that can ameliorate these challenges. This book offers O&M specialists and other professionals information and strategies to improve the mobility of this population, thus improving the quality of their lives and that of their family members. Changes in vision rehabilitation service delivery for older adults will occur as new medical conditions and treatments arise, new technologies are developed, and new laws are passed. To best serve older clients with vision loss, the field of O&M will want to be at the forefront of these developments.

References

Agency for Healthcare Research and Quality. (2004). *Vision rehabilitation for elderly individuals with low vision or blindness. Technology assessment.* Rockville, MD: U.S. Department of Health and Human Services, Centers for Medicare and Medicaid Services.

Associate for Education and Rehabilitation of the Blind and Visually Impaired. (2014, September). *Orientation and mobility division update.* Alexandria, VA: Author.

De l'Aune, W. R. (1980). Research and the mobility specialist. In R. L. Welsh & B. B. Blasch (Eds.), *Foundations of orientation and mobility* (pp. 653–662). New York: American Foundation for the Blind.

Farquhar, C., Lowe, J. I., & Campbell, J. W. (2007). Trends in aging funding and current areas of foundation interest. *Generations, 31*(2), 50–53.

LaGrow, S., Alpass, F., Stephens, C., & Towers, A. (2011). Factors affecting perceived quality of older persons with self-reported visual disability. *Quality of Life Research, 20*(3), 407–413.

National Aging and Vision Network Work Group. (1999, March). *Report from the Josephine L. Taylor Leadership Institute 1999.* Report presented at the annual Josephine L. Taylor Leadership Institute, Washington, DC.

National Eye Institute. (2012). *Vision research: Needs, gaps, and opportunities* (Research report). Bethesda, MD: U.S. Department of Health and Human Services, National Institutes of Health. Retrieved from https://www.nei.nih.gov/sites/default/files/nei-pdfs/VisionResearch2012.pdf

Orr, A. L. (1998). *Issues in aging and vision: A curriculum for university programs and in-service training.* New York: AFB Press.

Orr, A. L., & Rogers, P. (2001). Development of vision rehabilitation services for older people who are visually impaired: A historical perspective. *Journal of Visual Impairments & Blindness, 95*(11), 669–689.

Orr, A. L., & Rogers, P. (2003). *Self-advocacy skills training for older individuals who are visually impaired* [Training manual]. New York: AFB Press.

Orr, A. L., & Rogers, P. (2006). *Aging and vision loss: A handbook for families.* New York: AFB Press.

Orr, A. L., Scott, J., & Rogers, P. A. (2005). *The national agenda on vision and aging, 1998–2005: Report to the field.* New York: AFB Press.

Plouffe, L., & Kalache, A. (2010). Towards global age-friendly cities: Determining urban features that promote active aging. *Journal of Urban Health, 87*(5), 733–739.

Sauerburger, D. (n.d.). *An introduction to orientation and mobility skills.* New York: American Foundation for the Blind, VisionAware. Retrieved from http://

www.visionaware.org/info/everyday-living/essential-skills/an-introduction-to-orientation-and-mobility-skills/123

Virgili, G., & Rubin, G. (2010). Orientation and mobility training for adults with low vision. *Cochrane Database of Systematic Reviews, 12*(5), CD003925.

Wall Emerson, R. S., & De l'Aune, W. R. (2010). Research and the orientation and mobility specialist. In W. R. Wiener, R. L. Welsh, & B. B. Blasch (Eds.), *Foundations of orientation and mobility: Vol. I. History and theory* (3rd ed., pp. 569–596). New York: AFB Press.

Welsh, R. L. (1980). Additional handicaps: Visually impaired older persons. In R. L. Welsh & B. B. Blasch (Eds.), *Foundations of orientation and mobility* (pp. 420–428). New York: American Foundation for the Blind.

Wiener, W. R., & Siffermann, E. (2010). The history and progression of the profession of orientation and mobility. In W. R. Wiener, R. L. Welsh, & B. B. Blasch (Eds.), *Foundations of orientation and mobility: Vol. I. History and theory* (3rd ed., pp. 486–532). New York: AFB Press.

Wiener, W. R., & Welsh, R. L. (1980). The profession of orientation and mobility. In R. L. Welsh & B. B. Blasch (Eds.), *Foundations of orientation and mobility* (pp. 625–651). New York: American Foundation for the Blind.

World Health Organization. (2007). *WHO age-friendly cities project methodology. Vancouver protocol.* Accessed August 7, 2009, from http://www.who.int/ageing/publications/Microsoft%20Word%20-%20AFC_Vancouver_protocol.pdf

Yeung, P., LaGrow, S., Towers, A., Alpass, F., & Stephens, C. (2011). The centrality of O&M in rehabilitation programs designed to enhance quality of life: A structural equation modelling analysis. *International Journal of Orientation & Mobility, 4*(1), 10–20.

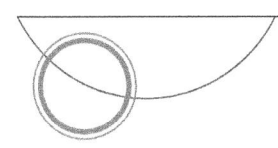

RESOURCES

*Compiled by Gabriella D. Davis, Project SASI
Technology Assistant, Texas Tech University, Lubbock*

The resources listed in this section represent a sample of the organizations, retailers, websites, and publications that provide information, guidance, and products helpful for the orientation and mobility (O&M) specialist who works with older adults.

The section on National Organizations contains organizations focusing on visual impairment generally, including professionals, organizations in the field, as well as those providing information and referral about specific visual conditions. Other listings include sources of products; videos; journals; and websites, which include resources for tactile graphics and technology; and specific resources for environmental adaptation and modification.

Although every effort has been made to provide accurate listings, such information is always subject to change, especially on the Internet. For more detailed listings of organizations and sources of products and services, see the American Foundation for the Blind's Directory of Services online at www.afb.org/directory.aspx.

NATIONAL ORGANIZATIONS
General Sources of Information and Referral

Academy for Certification of Vision Rehabilitation and Education Professionals (ACVREP)
4732 N. Oracle Road, Suite #217
Tucson, AZ 85705
(520) 887-6816
Fax: (520) 887-6826
www.acvrep.org

American Academy of Ophthalmology
655 Beach Street
San Francisco, CA 94109
(415) 561-8500
Fax: (415) 561-8533
customer_service@aao.org
www.aao.org

American Academy of Optometry
2909 Fairgreen Street
Orlando, FL 32803
(321) 710-3937 or (800) 969-4226
Fax: (407) 893-9890
aaoptom@aaoptom.org
www.aaopt.org

American Association of the Deaf-Blind
P.O. Box 8064
Silver Spring, MD 20907
Video phone: (301) 563-9064
aadb-Info@aadb.org
www.aadb.org

American Council of the Blind (ACB)
2200 Wilson Boulevard, Suite 650
Arlington, VA 22201-3354
(202) 467-5081 or (800) 424-8666
Fax: (703) 465-5085
info@acb.org
www.acb.org

American Foundation for the Blind (AFB)
2 Penn Plaza, Suite 1102
New York, NY 10121
(212) 502-7600 or (800) 232-5463
Fax: (888) 545-8331
info@afb.net
www.afb.org

American Optometric Association
243 N. Lindbergh Boulevard, Floor 1
St. Louis, MO 63141-7881
(800) 365-2219
www.aoa.org

American Speech-Language-Hearing Association
2200 Research Boulevard
Rockville, MD 20850-3289
(301) 296-5700
www.asha.org

Association for Education and Rehabilitation of the Blind and Visually Impaired (AER)
1703 N. Beauregard Street, Suite 440
Alexandria, VA 22311
(703) 671-4500
aer@aerbvi.org
www.aerbvi.org

Blinded Veterans Association
125 N. West Street, Floor 3
Alexandria, VA 22314
(202) 371-8880
Fax: (202) 371-8258
bva@bva.org
www.bva.org

CNIB
1929 Bayview Avenue
Toronto, ON M4G 3E8
Canada
(800) 563-2642
info@cnib.ca
www.cnib.ca

International Guide Dog Federation
371 East Jericho Turnpike
Smithtown, NY 11787
(631) 930-9000 or (800) 548-4337
Fax: (631) 930-9009
info@guidedog.org
www.guidedog.org
www.igdf.org.uk

National Blindness Professional Certification Board
101 S Trenton Street
Ruston, LA 71270
(318) 257-4554
Fax: (318) 257-2259
admin@nbpcb.org
www.nbpcb.org

National Center on Deaf-Blindness
345 N. Monmouth Avenue
Monmouth, OR 97361
(503) 838-8754
Fax: (503) 838-8150
info@nationaldb.org
www.nationaldb.org

National Coalition on Deaf-Blindness
175 North Beacon Street
Watertown, MA 02472
(617) 972-7768
Fax: (617) 923-8076
www.dbcoalition.org

National Federation of the Blind (NFB)
200 East Wells Street at Jernigan Place
Baltimore, MD 21230
(410) 659-9314
Fax: (410) 685-5653
nfb@nfb.org
www.nfb.org

National Library Service for the Blind and Physically Handicapped (NLS)
Library of Congress
1291 Taylor Street, NW
Washington, DC 20542
(202) 707-5100
TDD: (202) 707-0744
Fax: (202) 707-0712
nls@loc.gov
www.loc.gov/nls

Prevent Blindness
211 West Wacker Drive, Suite 1700
Chicago, IL 60606
(800) 331-2020
info@preventblindness.org
www.preventblindness.org

U.S. Council of Dog Guide Schools
c/o Pilot Dogs
625 West Town Street
Columbus, OH 43215
(614) 221-6367
Fax: (614) 221-1577

U.S. Department of Veterans Affairs
Blind Rehabilitation Service (117B)
810 Vermont Avenue, NW
Washington, DC 20420
www.va.gov
www.rehab.va.gov/blindrehab

Resources for Specific Eye Conditions

American Diabetes Association
1701 North Beauregard Street
Alexandria, VA 22311
(800) 342-2383
askada@diabetes.org
www.diabetes.org

The Association for Macular Diseases, Inc.
210 East 64th Street
New York, NY 10065
(212) 605-3719
www.macula.org

Foundation Fighting Blindness
7168 Columbia Gateway Drive, Suite 100
Columbia, MD 21046
(410) 423-0600 or (800) 683-5555
info@FightBlindness.org
www.blindness.org

Glaucoma Research Foundation
251 Post Street, Suite 600
San Francisco, CA 94108
(415) 986-3162 or (800) 826-6693
question@glaucoma.org
www.glaucoma.org

Macular Degeneration Support
3600 Blue Ridge Boulevard
Grandview, MO 64030
(816) 761-7080 or (888) 866-6148
director@mdsupport.org
www.mdsupport.org

Resources for Assistive Technology

Center on Disabilities, California State University, Northridge (CSUN)
18111 Nordhoff Street
Northridge, CA 91330
(818) 677-1200
Fax: (818) 677-4929
www.csun.edu/cod

Sponsors assistive technology training programs to expand the awareness of professionals and introduce newcomers to the disability field, and hosts the largest international conference focused on the field of assistive technology.

Closing the Gap, Inc.
526 Main Street
P.O. Box 68
Henderson, MN 56044
(507) 248-3294
Fax: (507) 248-3810
www.closingthegap.com

Serves as a practical resource covering the latest assistive technology news, how-tos and ever-changing technologies and implementation strategies.

Resources for Environmental Adaptation and Modification

Americans with Disabilities Act (ADA)
U.S. Department of Justice
950 Pennsylvania Avenue
Civil Rights Division
Disability Rights Section - NYA
Washington, DC 20530
(202) 307-0663 or (800) 514-0301
Fax: (202) 307-1197
www.ada.gov
Provides information about the ADA statute, ADA title II and III regulations, technical assistance materials, enforcement information, and general ADA information.

The Center for Universal Design
North Carolina State University, College of Design Campus
Box 8613
Raleigh, NC 27695
www.ncsu.edu/ncsu/design/cud
Evaluates, develops, and promotes accessible and universal design in housing, buildings, outdoor and urban environments, and related products. Develops publications and instructional materials and provides information, referrals, and technical assistance to individuals with disabilities, families, and professionals nationwide and internationally.

Environmental Geriatrics
Cornell University, Weill Medical College
1305 York Ave.
New York, NY 10021
www.environmentalgeriatrics.com
Develops geriatric-friendly environments such as retrofitting apartment dwellings to accommodate the needs of frail older adults as well as studies the impact of environmental design on health, independence, and function. Includes tips for home safety, modifications, and free online three-dimensional learning modules.

252 RESOURCES

Low Vision Design Program
National Institute of Building Sciences
1090 Vermont Avenue NW, Suite 700
Washington, DC 20005
(202) 289-7800
Fax: (202) 289-1092
www.nibs.org
Develops design principles and regulatory guidelines for creating safer and more accommodating environments for people with low vision.

Rehabilitation Engineering and Assistive Technology Society of North America (RESNA)
1700 North Moore Street, Suite 1540
Arlington, VA 22209
(703) 524-6686
Fax: (703) 524-6630
resna.org
Promotes the health and well-being of people with disabilities through increasing access to technology solutions and advances the field by offering certification, continuing education, and professional development; developing assistive technology standards; promoting research and public policy; and sponsoring forums for the exchange of information and ideas to meet the needs of our multidisciplinary constituency. Publishes *Assistive Technology* journal.

U.S. Access Board
1331 F Street NW, Suite 1000
Washington, DC 20004-1111
(202) 272-0080 or (800) 872-2253
TTY: (202) 272-0082 or (800) 993-2822
Fax: (202) 272-0081
www.access-board.gov
Promotes equality for people with disabilities through leadership in accessible design and the development of accessibility guidelines and standards for the built environment, transportation, communication, medical diagnostic equipment, and information technology and is a leading source of information on accessible design.

SOURCES OF PRODUCTS

The companies in the listings provided here are a sampling of those providing the products discussed in this volume.

Assistive Technology (Low Vision)

Access Ingenuity
4751 Hoen Avenue
Santa Rosa, CA 95405
(707) 579-4380 or (877) 579-4380
Fax: (707) 579-4273
customerservice@accessingenuity.com
www.accessingenuity.com
Offers a variety of assistive technologies from various manufacturers and an adjustable monitor arm stand for LCD monitors.

Ai Squared
130 Taconic Business Park Road
Manchester Center, VT 05255
(802) 362-3612
Fax: (802) 362-1670
sales@aisquared.com
www.aisquared.com
Manufactures screen magnification software and systems, and apps for iOS devices.

Clarix
2385 Cimarron Drive
Santa Clara, CA 95051
(408) 409-7333
Fax: (408) 625-7183
www.clarixusa.com
Manufactures video magnifiers, a screen reader (MagWin), a low vision magnifier, and free mobile magnifying apps.

Dolphin Computer Access
231 Clarksville Road, Suite 7
Princeton Junction, NJ 08550
(866) 797-5921 or (888) 519-4694
Fax: (609) 799-0475
InfoUS@YourDolphin.com
www.yourdolphin.com

Manufactures a digital Talking Book player, screen magnification systems, and a screen reader.

Enhanced Vision
5882 Machine Drive
Huntington Beach, CA 92649
(714) 374-1829 or (888) 811-3161
Fax: (714) 374-1821
www.enhancedvision.com
Manufactures video magnifiers.

Freedom Scientific
11800 31st Court N
Street Petersburg, FL 33716
(727) 803-8000 or (800) 444-4443
Fax: (727) 803-8001
www.freedomscientific.com
Manufactures handheld and portable video magnifiers, screen magnification and screen reading software, a DAISY player/recorder, and a portable scanning, reading, and magnifying device.

Innovative Rehabilitation Technology
13453 Colfax Highway
Grass Valley, CA 95945
(530) 274-2090 or (800) 322-4784
Fax: (530) 274-2093
Info@IRTI.net
www.irti.net
Manufactures digital Talking Book players and distributes a variety of products.

JBliss Low Vision Systems
737 Live Oak Avenue
Menlo Park, CA 94025
(650) 326-1235
jbliss.lowvision@gmail.com
www.jbliss.com
Manufactures optical character recognition systems and screen magnification systems. Also distributes a variety of screen readers and video magnifiers.

MagniSight
951 E. Fillmore Street
Colorado Springs, CO 80907
(800) 753-4767
Fax: (719) 578-9887
info@magnisight.com
www.magnisight.com
Manufactures video magnifiers and distributes a handheld video magnifier.

Your Low Vision Store
(800) 310-3938
www.yourlowvisionstore.com

A.T. Kratter & Co.
12062 Valley View Street, Suite 109
Garden Grove, CA 92845
(714) 799-3000

OVAC Assistive Technology
30111 Technology Drive, #110
Murrieta, CA 92563
(800) 325-4488

Infogrip, Inc.
1899 E. Main Street
Ventura, CA 93001
(800) 310-3938
Distributes a variety of video magnifiers and reading machines at its three locations.

Assistive Technology (Mobility)

Adaptive Technology Resources
1350 14th Avenue, Suite 3
Grafton, WI 53024
(800) 770-8474
Fax: (262) 375-6777
www.adaptivetr.com
Provides adaptive technology solutions for people who are blind or visually impaired, including software, cell phone applications, braille displays, notetakers, reading devices, and GPS systems.

HIMS, Inc.
4616 West Howard Lane, Suite 960
Austin, TX 78728
(888) 520-4467
Fax: (512) 837-2011
hims-inc.com
Manufactures the Braille Sense series of products, which feature built-in GPS receivers and electronic compasses.

HumanWare
1 UPS Way
P.O. Box 800
Champlain, NY 12919
(800) 722-3393
Fax: (888) 871 4828
info@humanware.com
www.humanware.com/en-usa/home
Manufactures and distributes a variety of products for people who are visually impaired, including the Trekker GPS and BrailleNote GPS software.

Sendero Group
739 Miller Drive
Davis, CA 95616
(888) 757-6810
Fax: (888) 757-6807
www.senderogroup.com
Develops GPS software and distributes GPS products and other devices and software.

Independent Living Products

The companies listed here distribute a wide range of independent living products, including braille products and supplies, adapted clocks and watches, computer software and access products, diabetes management products, kitchen and housekeeping items, labeling and marking products, lighting, low vision devices, mobility devices, personal care products, recreation and leisure products, talking products, telephones and accessories, and writing and reading devices.

Beyond Sight
5650 S. Windermere Street
Littleton, CO 80120
(303) 795-6455
Fax: (303) 795-6425
www.beyondsight.com

The Carroll Center for the Blind Store
770 Centre Street
Newton, MA 02458
(617) 969-6200 ext. 240
http://carroll.org/store

Future Aids, The Braille Superstore
33222 Lynn Avenue
Abbotsford, BC V2S 1C9
Canada
(800) 987-1231
Fax: (800) 985-1231
Sales@BrailleBookstore.com
www.braillebookstore.com

Independent Living Aids, LLC
137 Rano Street
Buffalo, NY 14207
(800) 537-2118 or (855) 746-7452
Fax: (516) 937-3906
www.independentliving.com

LS&S, LLC
145 River Rock Drive
Buffalo, NY 14207
(800) 468-4789
Fax: (877) 498-1482
www.lssproducts.com

Maxi-Aids
42 Executive Boulevard
Farmingdale, NY 11735
(631) 752-0521 or (800) 522-6294
TTY: (800) 281-3555
Fax: (631) 752-0689
www.maxiaids.com

Low Vision Products

Bausch & Lomb
1400 N. Goodman Street
Rochester, NY 14609
(800) 553-5340
Fax: (585) 338-6896
www.bausch.com
Manufactures a variety of handheld and illuminated magnifiers.

Bernell LV
4016 N Home Street
Mishawaka, IN 46545
(574) 259-2070 or (800) 348-2225
Fax: (574) 259-2102 or (574) 259-2103
info@bernell.com
www.bernell.com
Distributes a wide range of low vision and vision testing products and offers a line of vision therapy, visual rehabilitation, and behavioral optometry products.

Cocoons Eyewear
Live Eyewear
3490 Broad Street
San Luis Obispo, CA 93401
(800) 834-2563
Fax: (800) 654-7432
info@liveeyewear.com
www.cocoonseyewear.com
Manufactures UV absorptive filters designed for people with low vision and optical grade fitover sunglasses.

Designs for Vision
760 Koehler Avenue
Ronkonkoma, NY 11779
(631) 585-3300 or (800) 345-4009
infodvi@dvimail.com
www.designsforvision.com
Manufactures specialized optical products, including telescopes and microscopes for people with low vision.

Eschenbach Optik of America
22 Shelter Rock Lane
Danbury, CT 06810
(203) 702-1600 or (800) 487-5389
Fax: (888) 799-7200
www.eschenbach.com
Manufactures and distributes handheld, stand, and spectacle magnifiers; telescopes; video magnifiers; and a variety of low vision devices.

Good-Lite
1155 Jansen Farm Drive
Elgin, IL 60123
(847) 841-1145 or (800) 362-3860
Fax: (847) 841-1149
orders@good-lite.com
www.good-lite.com
Manufactures vision screening instruments and is the exclusive worldwide manufacturer of the LEA Test System.

NoIR Medical Technologies
6155 Pontiac Trail
South Lyon, MI 48178
(734) 769-5565 or (800) 521-9746
Fax: (734) 769-1708
noirsales@noirlaser.com
www.noir-medical.com
Manufactures sun filters.

Ocutech
109 Conner Drive, Suite 2105
Chapel Hill, NC 27514
(919) 967-6460 or (800) 326-6460
Fax: (919) 967-8146
www.ocutech.com
Manufactures bioptic low vision aids.

Richmond Products
4400 Silver Avenue SE
Albuquerque, NM 87108
(505) 275-2406
Fax: (810) 885-8319
www.richmondproducts.com

Manufactures and distributes a variety of vision assessment products, as well as prisms, lenses, and other products for ophthalmology and optometry.

Zimmerman Low Vision Simulation Kit
5700 Bunkerhill Street, # 2208
Pittsburgh, PA 15206
(412) 487-2818
Fax: 412-487-8365
lowvisionsimulationkit@yahoo.com
http://store.lowvisionsimulationkit.com
Distributes the Zimmerman Low Vision Simulation Kit.

Mobility Canes and Products

Advantage Canes
Revolution Enterprises, Inc.
12170 Dearborn Place
Poway, CA 92064
(800) 382-5132
Fax: (858) 679-5788
www.advantage-canes.com
Manufactures mobility canes and cane tips.

Aids to Independence Store
Society for the Blind
1238 S Street
Sacramento, CA 95811
(916) 452-8271
Fax: (916) 452-2622
Store@SocietyfortheBlind.org
http://societyfortheblind.org/store
Distributes cane tips and travel accessories such as cane holsters and cane repair tips. Also distributes braille products, household accessories, and writing aids.

AmbuTech
34 DeBaets Street
Winnipeg, MB R2J 3S9
Canada
(800) 561-3340
Fax: (800) 267-5059
www.ambutech.com

Manufactures and distributes a wide range of mobility canes and mobility aids.

HandiWorks
P.O. Box 19673
Kalamazoo, MI 49019
(888) 550-3063
Fax: (888) 412-8680
www.handiworks.com
Distributes dog guide gear, canes, and cane holders.

Independence Market
National Federation of the Blind
200 East Wells Street
Baltimore, MD 21230
(410) 659-9314 ext. 2216
Fax: (410) 685-2340
IndependenceMarket@nfb.org
nfb.org/independence-market
Supplies NFB white canes, as well as cane tips and tops, a support cane, a digital talking compass, a talking pedometer, writing aids, magnifiers, and medical devices.

Tactile Graphics Materials

American Thermoform Corporation
1758 Brackett Street
La Verne, CA 91750
(909) 593-6711 or (800) 331-3676
sales@americanthermoform.com
www.americanthermoform.com
Manufactures thermoforms that can be used for making tactile maps and other tactile graphics, as well as supplies, braillers, braille paper, and software.

American Printing House for the Blind (APH)
1839 Frankfort Avenue
P.O. Box 6085
Louisville, KY 40206
(502) 895-2405 or (800) 223-1839
Fax: (502) 899-2284
info@aph.org
www.aph.org

Distributes a variety of tactile graphics materials and kits that can be used for creating tactile maps and models, along with many other educational and daily living products and publications.

Duxbury Systems
270 Littleton Road, Unit 6
Westford, MA 01886
(978) 692-3000
Fax: (978) 692-7912
info@duxsys.com
www.duxburysystems.com
Manufactures the Duxbury Braille Translator for Windows and also provides other braille software.

InTouch Graphics
429 Winslow Avenue
Saint Paul, MN 55107
(347) 709-0845
joecioffi@intouchgraphics.com
www.intouchgraphics.com
Creates and produces tactile maps for university campuses, schools for the blind, museums, hotel lobbies, downtown areas of cities, camps, libraries, and other sites. Creator of ClickAndGo Wayfinding Maps, a narrative mapping service.

Perkins Products
175 N Beacon Street
Watertown, MA 02472
(617) 972-7308 or (855) 206-8353
Fax: (617) 926-2027
www.perkinsproducts.org/store/en
Distributes a variety of materials for creating tactile graphics.

ViewPlus Technologies
1965 SW Airport Avenue
Corvallis, OR 97333
(541) 754-4002
Fax: (541) 738-6505
www.viewplus.com
Manufactures braille embossers and software.

VIDEOS

American Foundation for the Blind. (2000). *What do you do when you see a blind person?* [DVD]. New York: Author. Available from www.afb.org/store

American Foundation for the Blind (Producer). (n.d.). *Orientation and mobility video* [Online video]. Available from: www.afb.org/info/programs-and-services/professional-development/experts-guide/orientation-and-mobility-video/1235

American Printing House for the Blind (Producer). (2007). *Reclaiming independence: Staying in the driver's seat when you no longer drive* [DVD]. Louisville, KY: Author. Available from: shop.aph.org

California Deaf-Blind Services (Producer). (2009). *Who's who: Orientation and mobility specialist* [Three-part online video]. Available from: www.cadbs.org/videos/o-m/

Texas Council for Developmental Disabilities (Producer). (2013). *Guide technique* [Online video]. Available from: www.projectidealonline.org/v/guide-technique

WEBSITES

AppleVis
www.applevis.com/
Offers multiple pathways to access and share relevant and useful information about Apple's range of Mac computers, the iPhone, iPad, and iPod Touch to empower the community of visually impaired users.

Dona Sauerburger, MA, COMS, Orientation and Mobility Specialist
www.sauerburger.org
Offers numerous articles, resources, tips, and teaching strategies about orientation and mobility from an expert in the field.

TactileGraphics.org
Lucia Hasty, Rocky Mountain Braille Associates
www.tactilegraphics.org
Provides basic information on production methods and techniques in the design and production of braille graphics and new products to assist in production of braille graphics; highlights on hardware, software, and upcoming opportunities for training and conferences.

Tactile Graphics Guidelines
Braille Authority of North America
brailleauthority.org/tg/web-manual/
Provides transcribers, educators, and producers with information about best practices, current methods, and design principles for the production of readable tactile graphics.

Tactile Graphics Resources
Texas School for the Blind and Visually Impaired
www.tsbvi.edu/component/content/article/107-graphics/3189-tactile-graphics-resources
Provides a list of tactile graphics resources, including tutorials on how to produce computer-generated line drawings for embossing and links to sources of tactile graphics materials.

VisionAware
American Foundation for the Blind
www.visionaware.org
Offers a wide range of information for adults with vision loss, their families, caregivers, health care providers, and social service professionals.

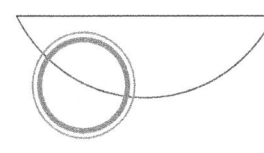

INDEX

Page references followed by *t* and *f* indicate tables and figures, respectively.

A

Academy for the Certification of Vision Rehabilitation and Education Professionals (ACVREP), 15, 242
accessibility
　ADA Standards for Accessible Design, 144–145
　Americans with Disabilities Act Accessibility Guidelines (ADAAG), 144
　built environment, 146–147
activities of daily living (ADL), 180. *See also* daily living skills, independent living
ACVREP (Academy for the Certification of Vision Rehabilitation and Education Professionals), 15, 242
ADA (Americans with Disabilities Act) of 1990, 143–146
ADA Standards for Accessible Design, 144–145
ADAAG (Americans with Disabilities Act Accessibility Guidelines), 144
adapting environment
　built environment, 143–151
　accessibility, 146–147
　Americans with Disabilities Act, 143–146
　barriers, 148–149
　certified aging-in-place specialists, 150–151
　defined, 143
　O&M assessment, 148
　universal design, 146–147
　creative process for applying themes, 158–161
　consistency theme, 153–155, 154f, 158–162
　contrast theme, 155, 156f, 158–162
　overview, 151–153
　texture theme, 155–156, 158–162, 158f
　transitions theme, 156–162
　independence in community living facilities, 197–199
　overview, 141–143
adaptive mobility devices (AMDs), 84, 85f
ADL (activities of daily living), 180. *See also* daily living skills, independent living
advocacy, O&M services, 241
African-Americans, 2
Agency for Healthcare Research and Quality, 10
age-related eye diseases (ARED), 4
age-related macular degeneration (ARMD), 2, 23–24
alignment, distance devices, 133
all-terrain tips, canes, 82f, 83
alternative living arrangements, 66
AMDs (adaptive mobility devices), 84, 85f
American Optometric Association, 190
Americans with Disabilities Act Accessibility Guidelines (ADAAG), 144
Americans with Disabilities Act (ADA) of 1990, 142–146
APH Tactile Graphics Kit, 126–127
aqueous, 23
ARED (age-related eye diseases), 4
Ariadne GPS for Apple devices, 124
ARMD (age-related macular degeneration), 2, 23–24

265

INDEX

Assessing the Learning Strategies of Adults (ATLAS), 206
assessments
  background, 34, 35f, 38–39
  built environment, 148
  functional, 37f, 39–40
  intake and functional assessment checklist, 36f
  low vision driver education training and, 195–196
assistance, requesting, 64–65
assistive listening devices, 130–131
assistive technology professional, 223
association strategy, room familiarization, 61
ATLAS (Assessing the Learning Strategies of Adults), 206
audio recorders, 130
audiologists, 14, 223
auditory compasses, 120
auditory maps, 128
auditory system. *See also* hearing loss
  central auditory processing disorders, 29
  conductive hearing loss, 27–28
  hearing aids, 30–32
  how hearing works, 26–27
  localization, 29–30
  sensorineural hearing loss, 28

B

backward navigation, walkers, 105, 105f
BADL (basic activities of daily living), 180. *See also* daily living skills, independent living
Balance Master Sensory Organization Test, 167
barriers
  built environment
    defined, 148
    hazards, 148–149
    obstacles, 148
  to collaboration among professionals, 228–230
  to safe driving for older adults, 191
basic activities of daily living (BADL), 180. *See also* daily living skills, independent living
Behavioral Risk Factor Surveillance System, 4
binoculars, 132
bioptic telescope system, 192–193
bioptics, 132
blended curbs, 157
Bonnet, Charles, 25
braille embosser, 127–128
built environment
  accessibility, 146–147
  Americans with Disabilities Act, 143–146
  barriers, 148–149
  certified aging-in-place specialists, 150–151
  defined, 143
  O&M assessment, 148
  universal design, 146–147
Business environment section, functional assessment, 39

C

cameras, 135
cane tips, 82f
  all-terrain tips, 83
  jumbo roller tips, 83
  marshmallow tips, 82
  metal glide tips, 82
  mushroom caps, 82
  pencil tips, 81
  roller ball tips, 83
  roller tips, 82–83
  wheel tips, 83
canes
  alternatives to, 85
  grips, 83–84
  long white cane
    overview, 80–81
    techniques for using, 62–64
    using with crutches, 96–97, 97f, 98f
    using with manual wheelchair, 112f
    using with support canes, 88–90, 90f, 91f
    using with walkers, 106–107, 106f, 107f
  support, 87–93
    overview, 87–88
    using as probe, 90–92
    using long cane with, 88–90
    using two canes, 92–93
CAPS (certified aging-in-place specialists), 150–151
capsule paper (swell paper), 127
cards and signs, 128–129, 129f
caregiving, 9
caretakers, 223
cars, negotiating, 62. *See also* driving
carts, 118–119, 118f
cataracts, 2, 22–23, 197
categorization strategy, room familiarization, 61
Caucasians, 2

Central auditory processing disorders, 29
certification of professionals, 242
certified aging-in-place specialists (CAPS), 150–151
Chang Tactile Graphics Kit, 126, 127f
Charles Bonnet Syndrome, 25–26, 196–197
climate, effect on navigation, 75–76
cochlea, 26
collaboration among professionals
  barriers to, 228–230
  defined, 214
  factors for success, 226–228
  interdisciplinary team model, 219
  multidisciplinary team model, 218
  overview, 213
  roles and responsibilities of rehabilitation team members, 221–222, 226
  settings, 216–218
  team strategies, 214
  transdisciplinary team model, 219–221
color and contrast, 199
color vision impairment, driving and, 191
communication
  devices for
    assistive listening devices, 130–131
    audio recorders, 130
    cards and signs, 128–129, 129f
    pads and markers, 130
    voice amplifiers, 130
  emergency preparedness, 201
  importance of, 47–48
  solicitation of aid, 64–65
community living facilities, independence in
  environmental modification, 197–199
  fire safety, 199–200
  overview, 196–197
comorbidity factors, 201
compasses
  auditory and talking, 120
  smartphone (digital), 120–121
  tactile, 119
  visual, 120
computer-generated maps, 124
conductive hearing loss, 27–28
consistency theme, environmental adaptation, 153–155, 154f, 158–162
constant-contact technique, cane, 63
contrast theme, environmental adaptation, 155, 156f, 158–162
convergent thinking, problem solving, 153
coping strategies, 5–6
counselors, 224
creative process, environmental adaptation
  overview, 151–153
  themes
    applying, 158–161
    consistency theme, 153–155, 154f, 158–162
    contrast theme, 155, 156f, 158–162
    texture theme, 155–156, 158–162, 158f
    transitions theme, 156–162
crutches
  gait patterns, 94
  guiding techniques with, 95
  overview, 94–95
  using as probe, 95, 96f
  using with long white cane, 96–97, 97f, 98f
curbs
  blended, 157
  as hazards, 148, 157f
  navigating with walkers, 102–106, 104f, 105f

D

daily living skills. *See also* independent living
  creating meaningful rehabilitation plans, 181, 183–184
  domains of independent living, 180–181
  driving, 188–196
    overview, 188–190
    psychological impact of not driving, 193–194, 196
    restrictions on, 190–193
  emergency preparedness, 200–203
    communication, 201
    overview, 200–201
    personal safety and health issues, 202–203
    support, 201–202
    travel, 202
  independence in community living facilities, 196–200

daily living skills *(continued)*
   environmental modification, 197–199
   fire safety, 199–200
   overview, 196–197
   learning theories and teaching methods, 206, 207
   life satisfaction and, 203–205
   low vision devices, 185–186
   overview, 179
   recreation, 186–188
demographics of older adults with vision loss, 2–4
depression, 6–7, 197, 200, 226
design, built environment, 146–147
diabetic retinopathy, 24–25
diagonal technique, cane, 63–64
digital (smartphone) compasses, 120–121, 121f
diplopia, 190–191
disability, defined, 144
distance devices, 133–135
divergent thinking, problem solving, 153
dog guides, 86
doorways
   improving visibility of, 152f
   negotiating, 52–53
driving
   overview, 188–190
   psychological impact of not driving, 193–194, 196
   restrictions on, 190–193
dual sensory impairment, 7–8, 31

E

ear, diagram of, 27f
electronic maps, 124
emergency preparedness
   communication, 201
   overview, 200–201
   personal safety and health issues, 202–203
   support, 201–202
   travel, 202
empowerment, O&M services, 241
environmental adaptation
   built environment, 143–151
      accessibility, 146–147
      Americans with Disabilities Act, 143–146
      barriers, 148–149
      certified aging-in-place specialists, 150–151
      defined, 143
      O&M assessment, 148
      universal design, 146–147
   creative process
      applying themes, 158–161
      consistency theme, 153–155, 154f, 158–162
      contrast theme, 155, 156f, 158–162
      overview, 151–153
      texture theme, 155–156, 158–162, 158f
      transitions theme, 156–162
   defined, 147
   independence in community living facilities, 197–199
   overview, 141–143
ethnicity, 3

exercise. *See also* recreation
   balance, 167–168
   chair exercises, 172
   endurance, 168
   exercise classes, 172
   exercise machines, 172
   fall prevention, 174
   flexibility, 168–169
   getting client started, 172–173
   overview, 165–166
   safety, 175
   sports, 171–172
   strategies for facilitating in older adults with vision loss, 173
   strength, 168
   tai chi, 169–171
   walking, 172
Eye Diseases Prevalence Research Group, 2

F

fall prevention, 174
falls, 64
Festinger, Leon, 204
fire safety, community living facilities, 199–200
flip maps, 128
FM (frequency modulation) technology, 146
forward navigation, walkers, 102
four-point alternate crutch gait, 94
frequency modulation (FM) technology, 146
functional assessment, 37f
   all environments, 39–40
   business environment, 39
   environmental considerations, 40
   home environment, 39
   residential environment, 39
   semi-business environment, 39

funding, O&M services, 240
furniture configuration, 199

G

gait belt, 54
gait patterns, crutch, 94
geography, effect on navigation, 75–76
glare reduction, 136–137, 199
glaucoma, 2, 22, 23, 197
Global Positioning System (GPS) receivers, 121–123
golf grips, cane, 84
GPS (Global Positioning System) receivers, 121–123
graphics mode on braille embosser, 127–128
guiding techniques
    crutches, 95
    grip for human guide for client support, 51f
    grip for human guide for client with balance issues, 50f
    narrow passageways, 52
    negotiating doors, 52–53
    overview, 48–51
    reversing directions, 51–52
    stairs, 53–54
    transferring sides, 52
    walkers, 101–102
    wheelchairs, 113–115, 114f

H

handheld magnifiers, 131f, 132, 135
hazards, built environment
    low ceiling, 162f
    overview, 148–149
    underside of stairs, 149f
health-related quality of life (HRQOL), 4
hearing aids, 30–32
hearing loss. *See also* auditory system
    conductive, 27–28
    sensorineural, 28
hemianopsia, 25
hip fractures, vision loss and, 3
Hispanics, 2
hospital walkers (standard walkers), 97–98
hospital wheelchairs, 110
HRQOL (health-related quality of life), 4

I

independent living. *See also* activities of daily living, daily living skills
    in community living facilities
        environmental modification, 197–199
        fire safety, 199–200
        overview, 196–197
    domains of, 180–181, 180t
indoor cane technique, 63–64
in-home attendant, 224
in-rhythm with cane, 88–89
in-step with cane, 88
Intake and Functional Assessment Checklist, 35f
    background and health, 34, 38
    functional vision observations, 38
    previous O&M instruction and travel routines, 38
    goals, 38-39
    current equipment, 39
intake assessment, 35f
interaural time difference (ITD), 29
interdisciplinary team model, 219

J

jumbo roller tips, canes, 83

K

knee walkers, 100, 100f

L

landmarks, room familiarization, 60–61
laser photocoagulation therapy, 24
LCD (liquid crystal display) screens, cameras, 135
learning theories and teaching methods, 206, 207
LED (light-emitting diode) screens, cameras, 135
life satisfaction, daily living skills and, 203–205
lighting, 199
liquid crystal display (LCD) screens, cameras, 135
living arrangements, alternative, 66
localization, 29–30
long white cane
    overview, 80–81
    techniques for using, 62–64
    using with crutches, 96–97, 97f, 98f
    using with manual wheelchair, 112f
    using with support canes, 88–90, 90f, 91f
    using with walkers, 106–107, 106f, 107f
low vision devices, 131-137, 185–186
    binoculars, 132
    bioptics, 132
    cameras, 135

low vision devices *(continued)*
   handheld magnifiers, 131f, 132, 135
   monocular telescopes, 131–132, 131f
   sunwear, 135–137
   video cameras, 135
   video magnifiers, 135
low vision services, 185–186
low vision specialists, 224–225
low vision therapists, 15, 182, 223
lower protective technique, 57

M

magnifiers, 131f, 132, 135
manual wheelchairs, 111t, 112–113, 112f
maps
   auditory, 128
   computer-generated, 124
   electronic, 124
   flip, 128
   overview, 123–124
   tactile, 124–128
marshmallow tips, canes, 82, 82f
medical walkers (standard walkers), 97–98
metal glide tips, canes, 82, 82f
mobility
   defined, 9
   quality of life and, 239
modifying environment
   built environment, 143–151
      accessibility, 146–147
      Americans with Disabilities Act, 143–146
      barriers, 148–149
      certified aging-in-place specialists, 150–151
      defined, 143
      O&M assessment, 148
      universal design, 146–147
   creative process for applying themes, 158–161
      consistency theme, 153–155, 154f, 158–162
      contrast theme, 155, 156f, 158–162
      overview, 151–153
      texture theme, 155–156, 158–162, 158f
      transitions theme, 156–162
   independence in community living facilities, 197–199
   overview, 141–143
modifying O&M techniques
   alternative living arrangements, 66
   cane skills, 62–64
   communication, 47–48
   guiding techniques, 48–54
      crutches, 95
      narrow passageways, 52
      negotiating doors, 52–53
      overview, 48–51
      reversing directions, 51–52
      stairs, 53–54
      transferring sides, 52
      walkers, 101–102
      wheelchairs, 113–115, 114f
   negotiating cars, 62
   overview, 45–47
   room familiarization, 60–61
   safety concerns, 64–65
      falls, 64
      personal safety, 65
      solicitation of aid, 64–65
   search patterns, 59–60
   seating, 58–59
   self-protective techniques, 54–57
      lower protective technique, 57
      upper protective technique, 54–57
   trailing, 57–58
monocular telescopes, 131–132, 131f
multidisciplinary team model, 218
mushroom caps, canes, 82, 82f

N

narrow passageways, guiding techniques for, 52
National Agenda on Vision and Aging, 240
National Blindness Professionals Certification Board (NSPCB), 242
National Eye Institute (NEI), 236, 238–239
National Institute on Aging, 167
negative stereotypes of persons with visual impairments, 5
NEI (National Eye Institute), 236, 238–239
neurological considerations for vision loss, 25
neuropathy, 33
NFB-style canes, 83–84
NSPCB (National Blindness Professionals Certification Board), 242

O

O&M services
  advocacy and empowerment, 241
  benefits of instruction, 9–10
  certification of professionals providing, 242
  effectiveness, 10–11
  funding, 240
  personnel preparation, 240–241
  provision of, 11–12
  public education, 241–242
  research, 236, 238–239
  response to challenges to provision of for older adults with vision loss, 237t–238t
  transportation, 12
O&M specialists
  collaborating with rehabilitation professionals, 13–15, 216
  low vision therapists, 15, 182, 223
  suggested responses to challenge of providing O&M services for older adults, 237t–238t
  teaching daily living skills, 182
obstacles, built environment, 148
occupational therapists, 14, 182–183, 224
ocular disorders
  age-related macular degeneration, 23–24
  cataracts, 22–23
  Charles Bonnet Syndrome, 25–26
  diabetic retinopathy, 24–25
  glaucoma, 23
  neurological considerations for vision loss, 25
older adults with vision loss
  demographics and trends among, 2–4
  effects of caregiving on family members, 9
  effects of vision loss experience, 5
  O&M services
    benefits of instruction, 9–10
    effectiveness, 10–11
    provision of, 11–12
    transportation, 12
  overview, 1–2
  psychological factors, 4–7
  psychological impact of dual sensory impairment, 7–8
olfactory system (sense of smell), 32–33
ophthalmologists, 224
optical devices. *See* low vision devices
optometrists, 224
orientation, defined, 9
orientation and mobility services. *See* O&M services
orientation and mobility specialists. *See* O&M specialists
orthopedic equipment
  carts, 118–119
  crutches, 94–97
  overview, 86–87
  support canes, 87–93
  walkers, 97–107
  wheelchairs, 107–118

P

pads and markers, 130
pencil tips, canes, 81, 82f
peripheral neuropathy, 33
personal safety, 65
personal sound amplifying product, 32
personnel preparation, O&M services, 240–241
physiatrists, 225
physical therapists, 14, 183, 225
physicians, 13, 225
point of interest (POI), GPS, 122
poverty, vision loss and, 3
power wheelchairs, 110, 111t
prefocusing, distance devices, 133
presbycusis, 28
probe
  using crutches as, 95, 96f
  using support cane as, 90–92, 92f
problem solving, environmental adaptation, 151–153
professionals, rehabilitation, 231. *See also* O&M specialists
  assistive technology professional, 223
  audiologists, 14, 223
  caretakers, 223
  collaboration among
    barriers, 228–230
    defined, 214
    factors for success, 226–228
    interdisciplinary team model, 219
    multidisciplinary team model, 218
    overview, 213

professionals (continued)
  roles and responsibilities of rehabilitation team members, 221–222, 226
  settings, 216–218
  team strategies, 214
  transdisciplinary team model, 219–221
 counselors, 224
 establishing rapport and trust with clients, 46–47
 in-home attendant, 224
 low vision driver education training and assessment, 195–196
 low vision specialists, 224–225
 low vision therapists, 15, 182, 223
 O&M specialists, 182
 occupational therapists, 14, 182–183, 224
 ophthalmologists, 224
 optometrists, 224
 orientation and mobility specialist, 223
 physiatrists, 225
 physical therapists, 14, 183, 225
 physicians, 13, 225
 psychologists, 224
 recreational therapists, 14, 225
 social workers, 225
 speech-language pathologists, 14, 225
 vision rehabilitation therapists, 15, 182, 223
psychological factors
 of aging, vision loss, and adjustment process, 4–7
 benefits of O&M instruction, 9–10
 of dual sensory impairment, 7–8
 psychological impact of not driving, 193–194, 196
 strategies for improving psychological and physical well-being, 8
psychologists, 224
public education, O&M services, 241–242

Q

quad canes, 88, 89f
quality of life (QOL)
 impact of visual impairment on daily living skills and, 203–205
 mobility and, 239

R

recreation
 adaptable activities for older adults with visual impairments, 189
 importance of, 186–188
recreational therapists, 14, 225
reducing shake, distance devices, 134–135
rehabilitation, creating meaningful plans for, 181, 183–184
rehabilitation professionals, 231. See also O&M specialists
 assistive technology professional, 223
 audiologists, 14, 223
 caretakers, 223
 collaboration among
  barriers, 228–230
  defined, 214
  factors for success, 226–228
 interdisciplinary team model, 219
 multidisciplinary team model, 218
 overview, 213
 roles and responsibilities of rehabilitation team members, 221–222, 226
 settings, 216–218
 team strategies, 214
 transdisciplinary team model, 219–221
 counselors, 224
 establishing rapport and trust with clients, 46–47
 in-home attendant, 224
 low vision driver education training and assessment, 195–196
 low vision specialists, 224–225
 low vision therapists, 15, 182, 223
 O&M specialists, 182
 occupational therapists, 14, 182–183, 224
 ophthalmologists, 224
 optometrists, 224
 orientation and mobility specialist, 223
 physiatrists, 225
 physical therapists, 14, 183, 225
 physicians, 13, 225
 psychologists, 224
 recreational therapists, 14, 225
 social workers, 225
 speech-language pathologists, 14, 225

Index

vision rehabilitation therapists, 15, 182, 223
rehearsal strategy, room familiarization, 61
research, O&M services, 236–239
reverse human guide technique, 101f
reverse walkers, 98–99
reversing directions, guiding techniques, 51–52
rigid canes, 81
rollators walkers, 99
roller ball tips, canes, 82f, 83
roller tips, canes, 82–83, 82f
room familiarization, 60–61
rural communities, assisting older adults with vision loss in, 69–78

S

safety concerns
    emergency preparedness, 202–203
    exercise, 175
    falls, 64
    fire safety in community living facilities, 199–200
    personal safety, 65
    self-protective techniques, 54–57
    solicitation of aid, 64–65
    wheelchairs, 108–109
scooters, 110, 111t, 112
search patterns, 59–60
seating, 58–59
self-protective techniques
    lower protective technique, 57
    upper protective technique, 54–57, 55f, 56f
sense of smell (olfactory), 32–33
sense of taste, 32–33

sense of touch (tactile system), 33
sensorineural hearing loss, 28
sensory changes with age
    assessments, 34–40
        background, 34, 35f, 38–39
        functional, 37f, 39–40
        intake and functional assessment checklist, 36f
    auditory system, 26–32
        central auditory processing disorders, 29
        conductive hearing loss, 27–28
        hearing aids, 30–32
        how hearing works, 26–27
        localization, 29–30
        sensorineural hearing loss, 28
    ocular disorders, 22–26
        age-related macular degeneration, 23–24
        cataracts, 22–23
        Charles Bonnet Syndrome, 25–26
        diabetic retinopathy, 24–25
        glaucoma, 23
        neurological considerations for vision loss, 25
        overview, 21–22
    sense of smell, 32–33
    sense of taste, 32–33
    sense of touch, 33
Sewell Raised Line Drawing Kit, 124–125, 126f
sideways navigation, walkers, 104, 104f
smartphone (digital) compasses, 120–121, 121f

social comparison theory, 204–206
social interaction, dual sensory impairment and, 8
social workers, 225
socioeconomic status, vision loss and, 3
solicitation of aid, 64–65
speech-language pathologists, 14, 225
spirituality, as coping strategy, 6
sports for visually impaired, 171–172
sports wheelchairs, 110
spotting, distance devices, 134
stairs
    guiding techniques, 53–54
    as hazards, 148, 149f
standard walkers, 97–98
stereotypes of persons with visual impairments, 5, 46–47
stigma of blindness, 46
stroke, vision loss and, 25
sunwear
    frames, 136
    lens tints, 135
    opacity, 135–136
support canes
    overview, 87–88
    use of long cane with, 88–90
    using as probe, 90–92, 92f
    using two canes, 92–93, 93f
    using with long white cane, 90f, 91f
swell paper (capsule paper), 127
swing-through gait, crutches, 94
swing-to gait, crutches, 94

INDEX

T

tactile bumps (truncated domes), 144–145, 145f
tactile compasses, 119
tactile maps, 125f
   APH Tactile Graphics Kit, 126–127
   Chang Tactile Graphics Kit, 126, 127f
   defined, 124
   graphics mode on braille embosser, 127–128
   Sewell Raised Line Drawing Kit, 124–125, 126f
   swell paper (capsule paper), 127
   thermoform, 127
   Wheatley Tactile Graphics Kit, 126
tactile system (sense of touch), 33
tai chi, 169–171
talking compasses, 120, 120f
telescoping canes, 81
texture theme, environmental adaptation, 155–156, 158–162, 158f
thermoform, 127
tools and techniques. *See also* long white cane
   adaptive mobility devices, 84, 85f
   cane alternatives, 85
   canes
      long white canes, 80–84
      support, 87–93
   communication devices, 128–131
      assistive listening devices, 130–131
      audio recorders, 130
      cards and signs, 128–129
      pads and markers, 130
      voice amplifiers, 130
   compasses, 119–121
      auditory and talking, 120
      smartphone (digital), 120–121
      tactile, 119
      visual, 120
   dog guides, 86
   Global Positioning System (GPS) receivers, 121–123
   low vision devices, 131–137
      binoculars, 132
      bioptics, 132
      cameras, 135
      handheld magnifiers, 132, 135
      monocular telescopes, 131–132
      sunwear, 135–137
      video cameras, 135
      video magnifiers, 135
   maps, 123–128
      auditory, 128
      computer-generated, 124
      electronic, 124
      flip, 128
      overview, 123–124
      tactile, 124–128
   orthopedic equipment, 86–119
      carts, 118–119
      crutches, 94–97
      overview, 86–87
      support canes, 87–93
      walkers, 97–107
      wheelchairs, 107–118
   overview, 79–80
tracing, distance devices, 134
tracking, distance devices, 134
trailing technique, 57–58
transdisciplinary team model, 219–221
transferring sides, guiding techniques, 52
transitions theme, environmental adaptation, 156–162
transport wheelchairs, 110
transportation, 12
travel, emergency preparedness, 202
trends among older adults with vision loss, 2–4
truncated domes (tactile bumps), 144–145, 145f
two-point alternate crutch gait, 94
two-point touch technique, cane, 63

U

universal design, built environment, 146–147
upper protective technique, 54–57, 55f, 56f

V

vibrotactile feedback, canes, 81
video cameras, 135
video magnifiers, 135
Vision Impairment Services Outpatient Rehabilitation (VISOR) program, 217
Vision Rehabilitation for Elderly Individuals with Low Vision or Blindness study, 10, 239
vision rehabilitation therapists, 15, 182, 223
Vision Research: Needs, Gaps, and Opportunities report, 236

VISOR (Vision Impairment Services Outpatient Rehabilitation) program, 217
visual compasses, 120
visualization strategy, room familiarization, 61
visual system, 22. *See also* ocular disorders
vitrectomy, 24
voice amplifiers, 130

W

Walker Waltz technique, 102, 103
walkers
    guiding techniques, 101–102
    knee, 100, 100f
    navigating curbs, 102–106, 104f, 105f
    reverse, 98–99
    rollators, 99
    standard, 97–98
    using with long white cane, 106–107, 106f, 107f
    walker waltz technique, 103
walking in step, cane, 63
weather, effect on navigation, 75–76
Wheatley Tactile Graphics Kit, 126
wheel tips, canes, 82f, 83
wheelchairs
    guiding techniques, 113–115, 114f
    hospital and transport, 110
    manual, 111t, 112–113
    navigating tight spaces and turns, 115, 116f, 117f, 118
    overview, 107
    power, 110, 111t
    safety, 108–109
    scooters, 110, 111t, 112
    sports, 110
    using with long white cane, 115
white cane. *See* long white cane
WHO (World Health Organization), 240